SOUTH MANCHESTER
INTENSIVE CARE UNIT

D0540980

Fundamentals of Anaesthesia and Acute Medicine

Pharmacology of the Critically Ill

Edited by

Gilbert Park

Director of Intensive Care, Consultant in Anaesthesia, John Farman Intensive Care Unit, Addenbrooke's Hospital, Cambridge

Maire Shelly

Consultant in Anaesthesia and Intensive Care, Intensive Care Unit, Withington Hospital, Manchester

SOUTH MANCHESTER
INTENSIVE CARE UNIT

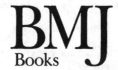

BMJ
Books

Cover image depicts the organic structure of morphine.

© BMJ Books 2001

All rights reserved. No part of this publication may be reproduced,
stored in a retrieval system, or transmitted, in any form or by any means,
electronic, mechanical, photocopying, recording and/or otherwise,
without the prior written permission of the publishers.

First published in 2001
by the BMJ Publishing Group, BMA House,
Tavistock Square, London WC1H 9JR

www.bmjbooks.com

British Library Cataloguing in Publication Data
A catalogue record for this book is available from the British Library

ISBN 0-7279-1221-6

Typeset by Phoenix Photosetting, Chatham, Kent
Printed and bound by J W Arrowsmith Ltd, Bristol

Contents

To those who have inspired us to look in directions
we might otherwise have missed.

Contributors

Bruno Bissonnette
Professor of Anaesthesia, Director, Divisions of Neurosurgical and Anaesthesia and Cardiovascular Anaesthesia Research, Department of Anaesthesia, The Hospital for Sick Children, University of Toronto, Toronto, Ontario, Canada

René Chioléro
Department of Anaesthesiology and Intensive Care, Centre Hospitalier Universitaire Vaudois, University of Lausanne, Lausanne, Switzerland

Geoffrey J Dobb
Intensive Care Unit and Department of Medicine, University of Western Australia, Royal Perth Hospital, Perth, Australia

Felicity Hawker
Director, Intensive Care Unit, Cabrini Hospital, Malvern, Victoria, Australia

Jean-Pierre Mustaki
Department of Anaesthesiology and Neurosurgery, Centre Hospitalier Universitaire Vaudois, University of Lausanne, Lausanne, Switzerland

Catherine O'Malley
Senior Registrar, Department of Anaesthesia and Intensive Care Medicine, Mater Hospital, Dublin, Ireland

Gilbert Park
Director of Intensive Care, Consultant in Anaesthesia, John Farman Intensive Care Unit, Addenbrooke's Hospital, Cambridge, UK

Dermot Phelan
Consultant in Anaesthesia and Intensive Care Medicine, Mater Hospital, Dublin, Ireland

Barbara J Pleuvry
Senior Lecturer in Anaesthesia and Pharmacology, University of Manchester, Manchester, UK

JW Sear
Reader in Anaesthetics, Nuffield Department of Anaesthetics, University of Oxford, John Radcliffe Hospital, Oxford, UK

Maire Shelly
Consultant in Anaesthesia and Intensive Care, Intensive Care Unit, Withington Hospital, Manchester, UK

Nerida A Smith
Senior Lecturer, Department of Pharmacology, University of Otago, Dunedin, New Zealand

Atul Swami
Department of Anaesthesia, Addenbrooke's Hospital, Cambridge, UK

Robert C Tasker
Consultant, Department of Paediatrics, Addenbrooke's Hospital, Cambridge, *and* Lecturer in Paediatric Intensive Care, University of Cambridge School of Clinical Medicine, UK

Wayne A Temple
Director, National Poisons Centre, Department of Preventive and Social Medicine, University of Otago, Dunedin, New Zealand

Robin J White
Specialist Registrar in Anaesthesia, John Farman Intensive Care Unit, Addenbrooke's Hospital, Cambridge, UK

Preface

This book is unusual in that it discusses how critically ill patients respond to the drugs they are given. It is not a book about the treatment of critical illness; many of these already exist. Rather than being just another textbook of therapeutics, its aim is to produce both knowledge and understanding of the underlying principles of pharmacology in the critically ill patient.

The reader might ask why such a book is necessary. There are two main reasons. First, the critically ill patients' condition is becoming more complex. The start of modern-day intensive care is generally taken as the polio epidemic in Denmark in the early 1950s. These patients had primarily respiratory failure, a single organ problem. Since then the number of simultaneous organ failures that are supported in the critically ill patient has increased. As well as respiratory failure, it is now common to support the kidneys, the cardiovascular system, the gastrointestinal tract, the liver, and the brain. As organs fail, so the pharmacokinetic processes of absorption, distribution, and elimination are affected. This changes the way drugs are handled by the body, often in ways that are difficult to predict. Multiple organ failure may also induce changes in the sensitivity of the target organ to a drug. For example, the encephalopathy of liver failure increases the sensitivity of the brain to sedative and analgesic drugs.

Second, just as the patients' condition has increased in complexity, so has their treatment. The number of drugs available to the clinician has increased dramatically since the early days of intensive care. Whereas, in the past, patients might have received a handful of drugs to treat and support their single organ failure, nowadays it is not uncommon for a patient with multiple organ failure to receive more than 20 drugs. This polypharmacy requires an understanding, not only of the pharmacokinetics of individual drugs in the critically ill, but also of how drugs interact when given to the same patient. Relatively few drugs are licensed for use in the critically ill patient; the costs and problems of the necessary research are prohibitive. It is essential then, that those prescribing drugs to critically ill patients have a full understanding of the problems that may arise from their administration.

No single book can describe all the possible pharmacokinetic changes or the potential interactions that may occur for every drug. There are simply too many. What we hope is that this book will give readers an insight into the complexity of the situation and some understanding of how to predict possible problems. To this end, we have invited a number of experts from around the world to describe the impact of major organ failures on how the critically ill patient deals with drugs. We emphasised to them that we wanted them to describe the principles of changes in pharmacology with organ failure, not how to treat organ failure. Each chapter has examples of treatments but these are meant to illustrate the concepts rather than provide comprehensive regimens.

The first chapters describe the fundamental principles of pharmacology: the pharmacokinetics of drugs, how they act and how drug receptors work. The second section of the book describes the effect of individual organ system failures on these fundamental principles. We are grateful to the authors of these chapters since literature with this emphasis is difficult to find; indeed, it usually does not exist. The final chapter of the book puts theory into practice, with a short chapter on how to prescribe drugs safely. The main author of this chapter is a trainee in intensive care medicine. We hope this contribution has produced a fresh and unbiased outlook on the subject and provided an approach for the future.

Gilbert Park
Cambridge

Maire Shelly
Manchester

1: Basic pharmacology

WAYNE A TEMPLE, NERIDA A SMITH

What a drug is

A drug in the modern sense, is any substance which affects normal bodily function at the cellular level. This is a very broad definition, as almost any substance will in some way at some level affect biological processes. Paracelsus (1493–1541) recognised this and wrote: "All things are poisons and there is nothing that is harmless; the dose alone decides that something is no poison." It is therefore necessary to know whether the amount of substance at its site of action is sufficient or excessive before deciding whether a chemical is a drug or poison.

Most drugs are effective because they bind to particular target proteins including enzymes, carriers, ion channels or receptors. For a drug to be useful as a therapeutic tool it must show a high degree of biological specificity. Small structural changes in the drug may lead to a change in biological response and these drugs are termed "structurally specific". Conversely, drugs such as gaseous anaesthetics are designated as "structurally non-specific" because small structural changes do not lead to changes in the biological effect. The activity of these drugs is related to the ratio of the partial vapour pressure of the substance in air and the vapour pressure of the substance (Ferguson's principle). Structurally non-specific drugs are generally active only in high concentration, whereas structurally specific drugs may produce a biological response at very low concentrations.

The biological properties of a drug are a function of its physicochemical parameters, such as solubility, lipophilicity, electronic effects, ionisation and stereochemistry. Structurally specific drugs interact with specific targets, forming a drug–receptor complex which may be stabilised by various forces (covalent bonding, ionic interactions, ion–dipole and dipole–dipole interactions, hydrogen bonding, charge transfer interactions, hydrophobic interactions and van der Waals interactions).

Covalent bonding is the strongest possible interaction and is of interest mainly in chemotherapy where it is desirable to have a drug which acts selectively on the target, to form an irreversible complex with its receptor so that the drug may exert its toxic action for an extended period. Unfortunately, for drugs to react covalently, this requires an increase in reactivity and consequently the desired selectivity may be lost. Non-covalent interactions are generally weak and several types of interactions may be involved in the drug–receptor complex. An electrostatic attraction, for example, may be due to an ion–ion, an ion–dipole or a dipole–dipole interaction.

Acetylcholine is an example of a molecule that can undergo an ionic reaction. The greater electronegativity of atoms such as oxygen, nitrogen, sulphur, and halogens relative to that of carbon, results in electronic dipoles for drugs containing a carbon-electronegative atom bond. Hence, the dipoles in a drug may be attracted by ions or other dipoles in the receptor. Similarly, hydrogen bonds are a type of dipole–dipole interaction formed between the proton of a group containing a hydrogen-electronegative atom (N, O or F) bond, and other electronegative atoms containing a pair of non-bonded electrons.

The ionisation state of a drug may have a marked effect on both its drug–receptor interaction and partition coefficient. Many drug molecules are weak acids or bases and can therefore exist in both unionised and ionised forms, the ratio of the two forms varying with pH. At physiological pH (pH 7·4), acidic groups such as carboxylic acid groups will be deprotonated to the carboxylate anion form. Similarly, basic groups, such as amines, will be protonated to the cationic form. Most alkaloids which act as local anaesthetics, neuroleptics and barbiturates have pK_a values between 6 and 8 such that both neutral and cationic forms are present at physiological pH. This may allow them to penetrate membranes in the neutral form and exert their biological action in the ionic form.

Chirality

Approximately 56% of drugs currently in use are chiral compounds, and 88% of these chiral synthetic drugs are used therapeutically as racemates. A chiral centre is formed when a carbon or quarternary nitrogen atom is connected to four different atoms. A molecule with one chiral centre is then present in one of two possible configurations termed enantiomers. These enantiomers have identical physical and chemical properties, but rotate polarised light in opposite directions. They are commonly referred to as optical isomers and are non-superimposable mirror images of each other (Figure 1.1).

One of these isomers rotates a beam of plane polarised light in a counterclockwise direction and is defined as the levorotatory or *l* enantiomer, and the angle of rotation is defined as a negative (–) rotation. The other isomer rotates light in a clockwise direction and is defined as the dextrorotatory or *d* enantiomer, and the angle of rotation is defined as a positive (+) rotation.

The earliest method of distinguishing one enantiomeric form from another was by the sign of rotation, i.e. *d* and *l* or (+) and (–) forms. Unfortunately, this did not describe the actual spatial arrangement around the chiral centre, known as the configuration. Consequently, a convention

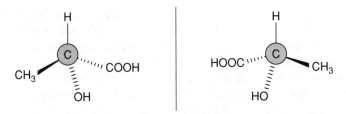

Figure 1.1   Lactic acid, an asymmetric molecule, and its mirror image.

was developed based on the sequence of substituents around the asymmetric centre.[1] A clockwise sequence is specified as R (Latin, rectus = right) or counterclockwise sequence S (Latin, sinister = left), to give R and S isomers.

The separation of enantiomers has an interesting background. In 1848 Louis Pasteur, using a hand lens and a pair of tweezers, painstakingly separated a quantity of the sodium ammonium salt of paratartaric acid into two sets of enantiomeric crystals. Because paratartaric acid (also known as racemic acid) was the first compound to be resolved into optical isomers (enantiomers), an equimolar mixture of two enantiomers is now called a racemate.

Most of the synthetic chiral drugs used in anaesthesia are administered as racemic mixtures (for example, the inhalation anaesthetics, local anaesthetics, ketamine), although some are single, pure enantiomers. Halothane, enflurane and isoflurane (Figure 1.2) contain a chiral centre and can exist as R and S isomers. Although the mechanism of anaesthetic action is not yet clearly understood, it has been shown that the pure enantiomers of chiral inhalation anaesthetic agents interact differentially with the CNS ion channels.[2]

Many naturally occurring compounds (formed by organisms or derived from plants) contain one or more chiral centres; however, their synthesis is usually stereoselective so that specific isomers are formed (e.g. *d*-tubocurarine, *l*-hyoscine and *l*-morphine), which are used therapeutically.

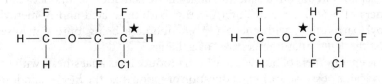

Enflurane   Isoflurane

Figure 1.2   Molecular structure of enflurane and isoflurane showing their chiral centres ($\star$).

An exception is atropine which occurs naturally as an *l*-isomer but is partly converted to its enantiomer during extraction and is consequently given as a racemate (*dl*-hyoscyamine). Since *d*-hyoscyamine has very little anticholinergic activity, the overall effectiveness of atropine is significantly reduced. The inactive or less active enantiomer of racemates was once considered an isomeric "ballast", but this certainly cannot be extrapolated to all racemic drugs. Today it is well recognised that changes in the enantiomeric makeup of chiral drugs may very significantly alter their pharmacokinetic properties and pharmacological and toxicological profiles.

Past practice was to develop racemates as drugs, either because their separation was difficult from a commercial perspective or the properties of the individual enantiomers had not been properly investigated. Now that new techniques are available for the large-scale separation of racemic mixtures or asymmetric syntheses to produce single enantiomers, there has been considerable effort directed at investigating their properties.

Atracurium is a complex mixture of 10 stereoisomers and is usually administered as the chiral mixture. Among these, *cis*-atracurium was isolated and its pharmacological properties were examined. This isomer offers clinical advantages over the mixture, principally due to the lack of histamine-releasing propensity and the higher neuromuscular blocking potency.[3]

Dobutamine is a racemate of two enantiomers both of which are positive inotropes. R(+)-dobutamine acts on β_1 and β_2 receptors, whilst S(–)-dobutamine acts on α_1 adrenoreceptors.[4] Since both isomers have similar desirable activities, this is an example where it is preferable to administer the chiral mixture rather than a single enantiomer.

Ketamine is a racemate containing equal parts of S(+)-ketamine and R(–)-ketamine. Several studies have been undertaken to compare the effects of the single enantiomers with the racemic mixture. The S(+) isomer of ketamine has about twice the analgesic potency of the clinically used racemic mixture and is about three times as potent as the R(–) isomer. The recovery phase was found to be shorter after S(+)-ketamine, compared with the racemate. The incidence of psychotic emergence reactions was thought to be due to the R(–)-ketamine from earlier human studies; however, subsequent studies have not demonstrated a consistently lower rate of psychic emergence reactions after S(+)-ketamine, compared with the racemate.[5] The separation of convulsant and anaesthetic activities occurs between the isomers of 5-(1,3-dimethylbutyl)-5-ethyl barbituric acid and N-methyl-5-propyl barbiturate, with the S-(+) enantiomers being pure convulsants whilst the R-(–) enantiomers are anaesthetics.[6]

The enantiomers of bupivacaine both produce local anaesthesia with S(–)-bupivacaine possessing a longer duration of action than the R(+)-enantiomer. The cardiotoxicity of bupivacaine may be due to R(+)-bupivacaine. Pharmacokinetic studies of these enantiomers has revealed that the enantioselective systemic disposition of bupivacaine can to a large extent be attributed to differences in the degree of plasma binding of the enantiomers.[7]

Labetalol, the mixed adrenoceptor blocker, is commercially available as equal proportions of four stereoisomers. Non specific β_1- and β_2-blocking activity is mainly conferred by the *R,R* isomer, while α_1-blocking activity is produced by the *S,R* isomer.[8] These examples given above serve to demonstrate that consideration of the stereoselective properties of enantiomers of chiral drugs may suggest therapeutic advantages over the use of racemates.

Some enantiomers have different therapeutic activities and as such may be marketed separately. For example, 2*S*,3*R*-(+)-dextropropoxyphene is an analgesic, and its enantiomer (–)-levopropoxyphene is an antitussive. The enantiomeric nature of these two drugs is also reflected in their US trade names, the former being marketed under the name Darvon® and the latter Novrad®.

In view of the modern technological advances which allow for the separation of racemate drugs, it is important that the individual isomers are fully evaluated for their pharmacological and toxicological properties to see if there are advantages in utilising one enantiomer in a particular therapeutic context. This has now been recognised by regulatory agencies involved with administering the control of medicines, such as the US FDA who released a policy statement for the development of new stereoisomeric drugs published in May of 1992.[9 10] This policy calls for identification of the isomeric composition of drugs with chiral centres and characterisation of their properties, including pharmacology, toxicology and clinical studies. It emphasises the need for drug manufacturers to develop quantitative assays for single isomers in *in vivo* samples early in drug development to facilitate the examination of the pharmacokinetic profile. Clearly it is important to evaluate not only new chiral drugs from this perspective but to study existing therapeutic racemates in order to optimise their clinical effectiveness.

Prodrug

A prodrug is a pharmacologically inert form of an active drug that must undergo transformation to the active form *in vivo* to exert its therapeutic effects. The primary purpose in forming a prodrug is to modify the physicochemical properties of the drug in order to influence its ultimate localisation. The conversion of prodrug to parent can occur by a variety of reactions, the most common being hydrolytic cleavage. Blood esterase can rapidly cleave many prodrug ester forms of hydroxyl or carboxyl groups of the parent drug. Biochemical oxidation or reduction processes may also be involved in the activation of the prodrug.

If the parent compound is insoluble, this can be modified by adding a water-soluble group which may be metabolically cleaved after drug administration. The local anaesthetic benzocaine is converted to water-soluble amide prodrug forms with various amino acids. Once administered, an amidase-catalysed hydrolysis occurs rapidly in the serum.[11] Diazepam, a benzodiazepine tranquilliser, is sparingly water soluble but can be produced *in vivo* from a freely soluble acyclic derivative that undergoes hydrolysis and spontaneous cyclisation to diazepam.[12]

5

A drug may be rapidly metabolised before it reaches the site of action, thus reducing its effectiveness or even rendering it inactive. Modification of the parent compound may block the metabolism until the drug reaches its target. Naltrexone (used in the treatment of opioid addiction), for example, undergoes extensive first-pass metabolism when given orally. Ester prodrugs of naltrexone substantially enhance its bioavailability.[13]

The slow and prolonged release properties of some prodrugs can confer several advantages, including the reduction in drug administration frequency, elimination of night-time administration, maximising patient compliance and reducing gastrointestinal adverse effects and toxicity. Haloperidol modified as the decanoate ester may be given intramuscularly as a solution in sesame oil. The antipsychotic activity of this prodrug lasts for about one month as compared with the short duration of activity if given orally.[14]

A drug may be toxic in its active form but if administered in a non-toxic, inactive form which converts to the active form only at the target site would have a higher therapeutic index compared with the toxic drug. Adrenaline, for example, used in the treatment of glaucoma, has a number of ocular and systemic side effects associated with its use. The dipivaloyl derivative of adrenaline, a prodrug, is almost as effective but has a significantly improved toxicological profile compared with adrenaline.[15] Site specificity is an important reason for prodrug design. In particular, selective delivery to the brain is a challenge for prodrug design. Only highly lipid-soluble drugs can cross the blood–brain barrier. Prodrugs with high lipid solubility can be used but may distribute to other regions and produce unwanted effects. L-Dopa (L-3,4-dihydroxyphenylalanine) reaches the desired target in the corpus striatum but also produces adverse effects in the peripheral tissues. Many of these side effects can be overcome by additional administration of an inhibitor of aromatic amino acid decarboxylase, such as carbidopa, that does not penetrate into the brain, but prevents transformation in the peripheral tissues.

Other prodrugs may be designed to overcome poor patient acceptability (e.g. unpleasant taste or odour, gastric irritation) or for formulation problems such as converting a volatile liquid form of a drug into a solid dose form.

Prodrugs then are typically designed with the purpose of maximising the binding of drugs to receptors. As outlined above, by altering the chemical structure of the active ingredient it is possible to enhance the pharmacokinetic properties and hence effect a promising drug transformation.

Pharmaceutical formulations

To facilitate the delivery of a drug by the most effective route, specific pharmaceutical formulations are prepared into forms such as tablets, capsules, syrups, creams, injections and so on. Specific properties of formulations may include the following:

- protect the drug from the atmosphere (oxidation, humidity), for example, coated tablets
- protect the drug from the acidity of the stomach, for example, enteric-coated tablets, injections
- conceal taste or smell, for example, coated tablets, capsules, flavourings
- provide time-controlled drug action, for example, controlled-release capsules and tablets, depot injections, transdermal patches.

Selecting the appropriate route, and hence the appropriate pharmaceutical formulation, for delivery of the drug is important. Cognisance needs to be taken of any changes that can affect the absorption of the drug. Increasing the pH of the stomach can affect the integrity of enteric coated tablets, causing the contents (usually of an irritant nature) to be released prematurely into the stomach. In the case of percutaneous delivery of local anaesthetics, toxicity has occurred following inadvertent applications to mucosal epithelia, or to denuded skin where the barrier to absorption is damaged or non-existent. A severe lignocaine intoxication occurred following application of a 5% topical formulation to painful, erosive skin lesions. The absorption barrier of the skin was no longer intact, and the patient displayed progressive toxicity culminating in fatal cardiorespiratory arrest.[16]

In addition to the active ingredient, a pharmaceutical formulation may contain non-therapeutic ingredients such as vehicles, thickeners, solvents, preservatives, sweeteners, flavours, stabilisers, colours, fillers, lubricants, plasticisers, humectants, propellants, disintegrants and suspending agents. Adverse reactions to these ingredients may be influenced by factors such as impaired excretion route, altered protein binding, membrane changes, chelation, enhanced or reduced absorption, duration of exposure and individual hypersensitivities. Solvents and preservatives in particular have been associated with adverse reactions.

Solvents

Solvents may be broadly classified into three types, polar, semipolar, and non-polar, based on their forces of interaction.

Polar solvents are made up of strong dipolar molecules having hydrogen bonding (for example, water and hydrogen peroxide). Semipolar solvents are made up of strong dipolar molecules but which do not form hydrogen bonds (for example, amyl alcohol and acetone). Non-polar solvents are made up of molecules having a small or no dipolar character (vegetable oil, mineral oil). Some solvents may fit into more than one class, for example, glycerin may be considered a polar or semipolar solvent even though it can form a hydrogen bond.

As a general rule, the greater the structural similarity between solute and solvent, the greater the solubility. Organic compounds containing polar groups capable of forming hydrogen bonds with water are soluble in water, providing that the molecular weight of the compound is not too great. Non-polar or very weak polar groups reduce solubility. Introduction of halogen

7

atoms into a molecule in general tends to decrease solubility because of increased molecular weight without a proportionate increase in polarity. The greater the number of polar groups the greater is the solubility of a compound, provided that the size of the rest of the molecule is not altered.

Water-miscible solvents suitable for pharmaceutical products are often employed to solubilise the active ingredient. There is a limited availability of low-toxicity solvents, and low molecular weight alcohols such as ethanol, propylene glycol and glycerin are commonly used. Higher alcohols such as the polyethylene glycols are also often utilised.

The effects of these solvents on the active drug may be difficult to predict and may include altering parameters such as the activity coefficient of reactant molecules, physicochemical properties, pK_a, surface tension, and viscosity, which may indirectly affect the reaction rate of chemical processes involving the drug.

In some cases the addition of a solvent may generate an additional reaction pathway, or there may be a change in the reaction mix. A solvent change may also change the stability of a compound, such as is found with the hydrolysis of barbiturates which is nearly sevenfold faster in water than in 50% glycerol.[17] The possibility therefore exists to stabilise a drug by the judicious choice of solvent; however, the limited availability of non-toxic solvents suitable for pharmaceutical products rather limits this approach.

Mineral oil is no longer used as a solvent for nasal preparations because of the danger of lipoid pneumonia and lipoid granulomata if small amounts are deposited into the small airways. Absorption of mineral oil is limited; however, it can be irritating and emulsified preparations may cause local granulomatous reactions.

Used topically, glycol is classified as a "minimal irritant"; propylene glycol is more irritating and sensitising. Polyethylene glycol when applied in large amounts to denuded, rather than intact, skin can be absorbed and undergo enzymatic depolymerisation to the systemically toxic mono-, di- and triethylene glycols. Generally, however, the small quantities used as solvents in parenteral formulations have not been associated with adverse effects, although care needs to be taken in patients with renal impairment and in infants. Local irritation may occur at the site of injection if amounts are excessive.

Glycerin is an effective parenteral solvent and in the usual quantities in parenteral formulations is free of toxicity. However, large quantities can cause hyperosmolality, and in turn intravascular haemolysis, haematuria, renal damage and hyperglycaemia.

Water for injection must be free of pyrogens and trace metals; the latter, although not inherently toxic, may alter the state of the active ingredient. Tonicity can be critical: aqueous intramuscular and subcutaneous injections that are much more painful than isotonic preparations; slow intravenous hypertonic solutions are well tolerated whilst hypotonic or aqueous preparations may cause haemolysis.

Preservatives

Preservatives have been defined by British regulatory agencies (The Preservatives of Food Regulations, SI 1982, No. 15) as "any substance which is capable of inhibiting, retarding or arresting the growth of microorganisms or any deterioration of food by microorganisms or of masking the evidence of any such deterioration". Additives such as spices, colourings and flavourings are specifically excluded from this definition.

Preservatives can be classified into three main classes:

- primarily microbial, for example, cetalkonium, cetylpyridinium, phenol, thymol, chlorocresol, chlorbutol, phenylmercuric nitrate/acetate, thiomersal, benzyl alcohol, benzoic acid, parabens
- antioxidants, for example, sulphites, ethylenediamine
- chelating agents, for example, ethylenediamine tetraacetic acid (EDTA).

As in the case of solvents, the quantities of preservatives in pharmaceutical formulations are generally too small to cause significant adverse effects. However, some individuals may be particularly sensitive to the preservative (most, but not all, of the preservatives), and greater exposures than originally intended can occur in neonates or following misuse.

Thymol is readily absorbed, and can discolour the urine. Exposure to excessive amounts has occurred following incorrect draining of vaporisers resulting in an accumulation of thymol sufficient to cause pulmonary oedema.[18]

Chlorocresol, used to preserve topical and parenteral formulations, has been associated with sensitisation, urticaria and contact dermatitis and anaphylactoid reactions having been reported.[19] Of perhaps greater significance have been reports of chlorocresol reacting in some way with suxamethonium, triggering malignant hyperthermia in susceptible persons. It is believed that a defect in the ryanodine receptor Ca^{2+} channel is implicated as one of the causes, and that chlorocresol enhances the Ca^{2+} release from the sarcoplasmic reticulum.[20]

Prolonged exposure to benzyl alcohol (used in concentrations ranging from 1 to 10%) can cause neurotoxicity, and intrathecal injections have resulted in paraplegia.[21] Benzyl alcohol is no longer recommended for use as preservatives for injectables in neonates, given the high dose per kilogram administered and the low tolerance of neonates, reflecting the underdeveloped pathway of oxidising benzyl alcohol to benzoic acid and then converting to hippuric acid for excretion.

Bronchoconstriction following inhalation of benzalkonium chloride used as a preservative in antiasthma nebuliser solutions has been reported on a number of occasions.[22,23] The commonly used concentration (0·01%) does not cause detectable damage when applied topically, although a 0·1% solution has been irritating when applied to the eye.[19]

The sulphite-type antioxidants can cause a variety of problems in intolerant subjects: gastric irritation, systemic respiratory circulatory collapse and central nervous system depression.[19] Seizures following intravenous administration of high-dose morphine containing sodium bisulphite as a preservative and the absorption of bisulphite from peritoneal dialysis solutions have been reported.[19,22,24,25] The sulphites are metabolised rapidly to the sulphate, which is excreted renally.

EDTA is poorly absorbed orally, is essentially unmetabolised and excreted via the kidneys as the calcium complex and has an affinity for metals much heavier than calcium, such as lead, iron and plutonium. Chronic use of EDTA has shown adverse effects resembling zinc deficiencies, which if not corrected can result in renal toxicity.[19]

How to measure drug concentrations

In practice, there is no advantage in measuring the concentration of a drug in a biological fluid if its biological effect can be easily monitored. For example, it is more pertinent to measure blood glucose rather than the blood levels of oral antidiabetic agents. Similarly, blood pressure monitoring may be more informative than measuring blood concentrations of antihypertensive agents. Plasma prothrombin time measurements may be more relevant than determining plasma levels of therapeutic agents used in anticoagulant therapy. However, there are several drugs for which blood concentrations have been shown unequivocally to provide clinically useful information. The narrow margin between therapeutic and toxic plasma levels for lithium is a prime example where it is essential to monitor the plasma concentration in order to adjust the dosage regimen.

A variety of analytical techniques are available for measuring drug concentrations in body fluids. The most important of these techniques are radioimmunoassay (RIA) and related types of analysis, various separation techniques involving chromatography and/or mass spectrometry with high sensitivity detector, and photometric and fluorimetric techniques.

RIA involves employing an antibody which binds specifically and with high affinity to the drug to be assayed. A radiolabelled version of the drug is mixed together with the drug and antibody and the resulting solution is then separated into antibody-bound and free material. A radioactive count of the free or bound fraction is then undertaken to determine the drug concentration (Figure 1.3).

Enzyme immunoassay (EIA) or enzyme-linked immunosorbent assay (ELISA) is a variant of RIA in which the label used is an enzyme rather than a radiolabel (Figure 1.4). The enzyme-coupled derivative of the drug to be analysed is prepared, by a covalent coupling reaction, and a standard amount is added to the assay mixture together with the antibody and drug. The amount of enzyme-coupled derivative that combines with the antibody will depend on the amount of drug in the sample. Usually, the enzymic activity of this bound fraction is much less than that of the enzyme-coupled derivative so that no separation is necessary and a simple (usually photometric) measure of enzyme activity in the mixture is then undertaken. The

10

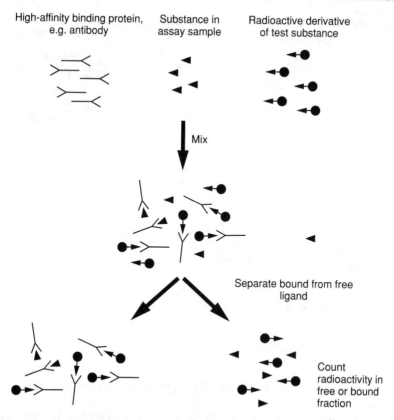

High-affinity binding protein, e.g. antibody

Substance in assay sample

Radioactive derivative of test substance

Mix

Separate bound from free ligand

Count radioactivity in free or bound fraction

Figure 1.3   The principle of immunoassay.

more drug that is present, the greater the amount of free enzyme-coupled derivative and the greater the enzymic activity. This type of assay is known as EMIT (enzyme-multiplied immunoassay technique). Generally the sensitivity of the immunoassays is extremely high and can work in the range 10^{-12}–10^{-14} mol.

Chromatographic techniques for separating substances combined with sensitive detection systems are the basis for many drug assay systems. Gas chromatography (GC) involves volatilising the sample and passing the gaseous medium through a narrow column of solid absorbent at high temperature in order to effect a separation of the components in the sample. The emerging substances can be detected by various detection systems including flame ionisation, electron capture and the most sensitive type, mass spectrometry (MS). The GCMS technique will permit samples containing as little as 10^{-15} mol of drug to be assayed.

High performance liquid chromatography (HPLC) is similar to GC but utilises a liquid rather than gas phase for separation of the sample.

11

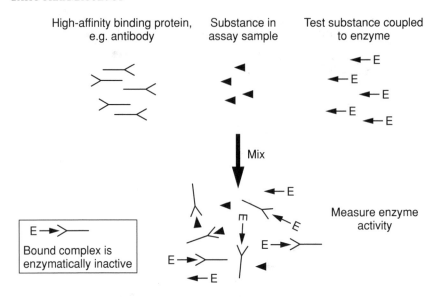

Figure 1.4   The principle of enzyme-linked assay.

Detection systems include UV and MS. HPLC is routinely used for many drug assays.

Spectroscopic methods, especially fluorimetry, provide highly high-sensitivity detector systems that can often be used in conjunction with HPLC separation.

Plasma (or serum) drug concentrations can be used to guide the treatment of individual patients if several parameters are known and include: the therapeutic range of plasma concentrations for the drug; the clinical pharmacokinetics for the drug; the timing of drug administration to the patient; details of other drug treatment.

Plasma and tissue concentrations of drugs are in equilibrium by the time drug distribution is complete. Most drugs circulate partly bound to erythrocytes or plasma proteins, the bound drug being in equilibrium with the unbound drug. It is the plasma (unbound drug) that is of particular interest in therapeutic drug monitoring. Unfortunately, measurement of unbound drug presents difficulties and drug monitoring mostly depends on measurements of plasma.

Only a few drug assays are of proven clinical value: aminoglycosides, digoxin, anticonvulsants (for example, carbamazepine, phenobarbitone, phenytoin), immunosuppressants (cyclosporin, tacrolimus), and a few others (for example, theophylline and lithium). However, there are several other drugs that are considered promising candidates for therapeutic drug monitoring, particularly when administration is for the long term and therapy is essential for patient survival or can produce severe side effects or both. Methotrexate is the only commonly measured drug (albeit by relatively few laboratories) used in cancer therapy; however, a number of drugs used in the treatment of haematological cancers are good candidates for therapeutic drug monitoring.[26] There is also recent evidence that the monitoring of the anti-acquired immunodeficiency syndrome agents zidovudine[27] and didanosine in plasma are useful clinically.

The timing of blood specimen collection for drug monitoring is extremely important. In general, it takes about five times the elimination half-time of a drug for its plasma concentration to achieve a steady state with a particular dosage level. For example, with digoxin, blood should be taken at least six hours after the last dose, when absorption and distribution are usually complete. Plasma concentrations of lithium should be measured on a specimen taken 12 hours after the last dose, as trough concentrations are particularly important for therapeutic control.

In cases of suspected intoxication such sampling is not feasible, but it should be kept in mind that concentrations obtained fairly soon post-ingestion may not be predictive of outcome.

The use of digoxin-specific antibodies in the management of digoxin overdose is another example where care must be taken when interpreting plasma drug concentrations. Antibody fragments affect commercially available digoxin assay kits which measure both the free (digoxin available for receptor binding) and total (free digoxin plus that bound to antibody) digoxin such that the serum digoxin concentration rises rapidly after antibody infusion, most of which is biologically inactive. Monitoring the patient's serum digoxin concentration after the administration of antibody is not possible until the antibody-bound digoxin is cleared from the blood, usually within five days in a patient without underlying renal failure. Newer, more accurate methods using ultrafiltration coupled with a fluorescence polarisation immunoassay are able to distinguish between free and bound digoxin, which is useful in the monitoring of patients.[28] Specific analytical methods are also required if active drugs and structurally closely related but nevertheless inactive compounds (metabolites) are to be differentiated. Specific methods are required for therapeutic drug monitoring, since results from methods that fail to differentiate between active drugs and related but inactive compounds are of limited value.

In some cases, metabolites may be pharmacologically more active than the parent drug. Morphine, for example, is metabolised primarily to two glucuronide metabolites, morphine-3-glucuronide and morphine-6-glucuronide, both of which have been reported to be pharmacologically active. Morphine-6-glucuronide has been shown to be a more potent analgesic than morphine;[29] thus it is important to be able to measure the plasma concentrations of morphine and its metabolites in order to more fully evaluate pharmacokinetic data derived from patients treated with morphine. Although there are a large number of assays available for the measurement of morphine (RIA, HPLC, GLC), there are relatively few assays capable of determining morphine and its glucuronide metabolites together.[30] It is therefore important for clinicians to ascertain what drug measurement options are available to them in order to decide the best practical option for therapeutic drug monitoring of their patients.

Summary points

- Most drugs are effective because they bind to particular target proteins including enzymes, carriers, ion channels or receptors.
- Drug enantiomers may differ considerably in potency, pharmacological activity and pharmacokinetic profile.
- A prodrug is a pharmacologically inert form of an active drug that must undergo transformation to the active form *in vivo* to exert its therapeutic effects.
- Specific pharmaceutical formulations are prepared into forms such as tablets, capsules, syrups, creams and injections to facilitate the delivery of a drug by the most effective route.
- Solvents may be broadly classified into three types, polar, semipolar, and non-polar, based on their forces of interaction. Their effects may be difficult to predict and may include altering the physicochemical and pharmacodynamic properties of the drug.
- The quantities of preservatives in pharmaceutical formulations are generally too small to cause significant adverse effects; however, some individuals may be particularly sensitive to the preservative and greater exposures than originally intended can occur in neonates or following misuse.
- A variety of analytical techniques are available for measuring drug concentrations in body fluids, including radioimmunoassay (RIA), chromatography, mass spectrometry, photometric and fluorimetric techniques. However, there is no advantage in measuring drug concentrations if the biological effect can be easily monitored.

1 Wainer IW. *Drug Stereochemistry. Analytical methods and pharmacology*, 2nd edn. New York: Marcel Dekker, Inc., 1993 : 25–34.
2 Polavarapu PL, Cholli AL, Vernice G. Determination of absolute configurations and predominant conformations of general inhalation anaesthetics: desflurane. *J Pharm Sci* 1993;**82**:791–3.
3 Nigrovic V, Diefenbach C, Mellinghoff H. Esters and stereoisomers *Anaesthesist* 1997;**46**:282–6.
4 Calvey TN. Isomerism and anaesthetic drugs. *Acta Anaesthesiol Scand Suppl* 1995;**106**:83–90.
5 Engelhardt W. Aufwachverhalten und psychomimetische reaktionen nach S-(+)-ketamin *Anaesthesist* 1997;**46**(Suppl 1):S38–42.
6 Downes H, Perry RS, Ostlund RE, Karler R. A study of the excitatory effects of barbiturates. *J Pharmacol Exp Ther* 1970;**175**(3):692–9.
7 Bum AG, van der Meer AD, van Kleef JW, Zeijlmans PW, Groen K. Pharmacokinetics of the enantiomers of bupivacaine following intravenous administration of the racemate. *Br J Clin Pharmacol* 1994;**38**:125–9.
8 Prichard BNC. Combined α- and β-adrenoreceptor inhibition in the treatment of hypertension. *Drugs* 1984;**28**:51–68.

9 Tomaszewski J, Rumore MM. Stereoisomeric drugs: FDA's policy statement and the impact on drug development. *Drug Dev Indust Pharm* 1994;**20**:119–39.
10 Rauws AG, Groen K. Current regulatory guidance on chiral medicinal products: Canada, EEC, Japan and US. *Chirality* 1994;**6**:72–5.
11 Slojkowska Z, Krasuska HJ, Pachecka J. Enzymatic hydrolysis of amino acid derivatives of benzocaine *Xenobiotica* 1982;**12**:359–64.
12 Hirai K, Ishiba T, Sugimoto H, Fujishita T, Tsukinoki Y, Hirose K. Novel peptidoaminobenzophenones, terminal *N*-(acylglycl)aminobenzophenones as open-ring derivatives of benzodiazepines. *J Med Chem* 1981;**24**:20–7.
13 Hussain MA, Koval CA, Myers MJ, Shami EG, Shefter E. Improvement of the oral bioavailability in dogs: a prodrug approach. *J Pharm Sci* 1987;**76**:356–8.
14 Deberdt R, Elens P, Berghmans W *et al.* Intramuscular haloperidol decanoate for neuroleptic maintenance therapy. Efficacy, dosage schedule and plasma levels. An open multicenter study. *Acta Psychiatr Scand* 1980;**62**:356–63.
15 Mandell AI, Stentz F, Kitabchi AE. Dipivalyl epinephrine: a new pro-drug in the treatment of glaucoma. *Ophthalmology* 1978;**85**:268–75.
16 Lie RL, Vermeer BJ, Edelbroek PM. Severe lidocaine intoxication by cutaneous absorption. *J Am Acad Dermatol* 1990;**25**:1026–8.
17 Thoma K, Struve M. Stabilization of barbituric acid derivatives in aqueous solutions. Part 1. Influence of hydophilic nonaqueous solvents on the stability of barbituric acid derivatives. *Pharm Ind* 1985;**47**:1078–81.
18 Euarby MR, Walker JE. HPLC of thymol in halothane BP and halothane vapourizer waste. *Br J Pharm Pract* 1984;**6**:373–4.
19 Weiner M, Bernstein IL, eds. *Adverse reactions to drug formulation agents. A handbook of excipients.* New York: Marcel Dekker Inc., 1989.
20 Tegazzin V, Scutari E, Treves S, Zorzato F. Chlorocresol, an additive to commercial succinylcholine, induces contracture of human malignant hyperthermia-susceptible muscles via activation of the ryanodine receptor Ca^{2+} channel. *Anethesiology* 1996;**84**(6):1380–5.
21 Saiki JH, Thompson S, Smith F, Atkinson R. Paraplegia folowing intrathecal chemotherapy. *Cancer* 1972;**29**:370–4.
22 Boucher M, Roy MT, Henderson J. Possible association of benzalkonium chloride in nebulizer solutions with respiratory arrest. *Ann Pharmacother* 1992;**26**(6):772–4.
23 Zhang YG, Wright WJ, Tam WK, Nguyen-Dang TH, Salome CM, Woolcock AJ. Effect of inhaled preservatives on asthmatic subjects. II. Benzalkonium chloride. *Am Rev Respir Dis* 1990;**141**(6):1405–8.
24 Gregory RE, Grossman S, Sheidler VR. Grand mal seizures associated with high-dose intravenous morphine infusions: incidence and possible etiology. *Pain* 1992;**51**(2):255–8.
25 Meisel SB, Welford PK. Seizures associated with high-dose intravenous morphine containing sodium bisulfite preservative. *Ann Pharmacother* 1992;**26**(12):1515–17.
26 Galpin AJ, Evans WE. Therapeutic drug monitoring in cancer management. *Clin Chem* 1993;**11**(part 2):2419–30.
27 Stretcher BN, Pesce AJ, Frame PT, Greenberg KA, Stein DS. Correlates of zidovudine phosphorylation with markers of HIV disease progression and drug toxicity. *AIDS* 1994;**8**:763–9.
28 Banner W Jr, Bach P, Burk B, Freestone S, Gooch WM 3rd. Influence of assay methods on serum concentrations of digoxin during FAB fragment treatment. *J Toxicol Clin Toxicol* 1992;**30**(2):259–67.
29 Hanna MH, Peat SJ, Woodham M, Knibb A, Fung C. Analgesic efficacy and CSF pharmacokinetics of intrathecal M6G in comparison with morphine. *Br J Anaesth* 1990;**64**:547–50.
30 Zuccaro P, Ricciarrello R, Pichini S *et al.* Simultaneous determination of heroin 6-monoacetylmorphine, morphine, and its glucuronides by liquid chromatography-atmospheric pressure ionspray-mass spectrometry. *J Anal Toxicol* 1997;**21**:268–77.

2: Pharmacokinetics and pharmacodynamics

GILBERT PARK

Every critically ill patient is given many drugs, some patients may receive up to 20 drugs simultaneously. Despite the frequent use of drugs, surprisingly little is known about their use in the critically ill. There is often an awareness that there may be an exaggerated response in say, the haemodynamic effects of a new sedative agent compared with its use during anaesthesia, but little else. The way new drugs are developed goes some way to explain this. Those destined for the critically ill are conceived on the laboratory bench, tried in healthy animals and then given to healthy volunteers. If they are tried in patients, then it is usually in patients with a stable form of a chronic disease. With this limited information drugs are then used in the critically ill. It should not be surprising that the use of these drugs in patients with very deranged bodily functions, often in combination with other drugs, result in unpredictable effects. This chapter aims to explain some of the mechanisms by which these effects occur.

Drug absorption

Unless a drug is given at its site of action, it needs to be absorbed into the blood and be transported to its site of action. Oral, intramuscular and the intravenous routes are the commonest when giving drugs to critically ill patients. However, other routes may also be used. For example, an inhalational route may be used for β-sympathomimetic drugs such as salbutamol and also for sedative agents such as isoflurane.[1,2] The rectal route, which is not subject to the same vagaries of absorption as the rest of the gastrointestinal tract, has been used for the administration of drugs such as paracetamol, that may not be available in a parenteral formulation.

Those drugs given enterally must pass through the gastrointestinal wall to enter the bloodstream. The absorption of drugs is affected not only by their formulation, resistance to gastric acid and intestinal enzymes, but also by motility and interactions with drug and food. How lipid soluble they are will also affect their absorption. Drugs exist in equilibrium between ionised and non-ionised forms. The degree of ionisation depends on the pK_a of the drug and the pH of the solution. The pK_a is the negative logarithm of the dissociation constant, and it is also the pH at which 50% of the drug is ionised and 50% is non-ionised. It is the non-ionised form of the drug that is lipid soluble and diffuses across cell membranes. The ionised form cannot cross membranes. Alcohol and chloral hydrate are non-ionised drugs which cross membranes freely.

Drugs absorbed from the gastrointestinal tract enter first the portal circulation and pass through the liver. Some drugs are extensively metabolised as they pass through the gut wall (isoprenaline) and the liver (lignocaine, propranolol). Because of this, they may not reach a concentration in the systemic circulation sufficient to exert a pharmacological effect. This is known as first-pass metabolism.

In the critically ill, the gastrointestinal tract commonly fails. This may be a problem if oral drugs are given during a period of gut stasis. Repeated, ineffectual doses may be given that then accumulate in the stomach. When gastrointestinal motility restarts, a potentially toxic amount of the drug may then be absorbed. Conversely, when there is gastrointestinal rush, drugs may not be absorbed. In addition, splanchnic blood flow is variable in the critically ill and this in combination with the stasis makes the enteral route for drugs unreliable.

The parenteral route avoids some of the problems associated with the enteral route. Intramuscular and subcutaneous injection does not completely overcome these problems. Both are subject to changes in blood flow in the critically ill patient. If there is a low blood flow (such as in shock), then the drug will not be absorbed. Again, potentially toxic doses of drugs can be given because they are repeated as the first dose appears ineffectual. When blood flow is restored, this large dose may then be absorbed. Direct intravenous injection overcomes all of the difficulties associated with other routes of administration. Because of this it is the commonest route used in the critically ill.

Drug distribution

Once a drug enters the systemic circulation it is distributed around the body. From there it penetrates tissues to reach its site of action. Several factors will affect the rate at which this happens. These include:

- the degree of protein binding
- the ability to diffuse across the endothelium, interstitial fluid, and cellular membranes
- blood flow to the organ concerned.

The volume of distribution (V_d) represents the apparent volume available in the body for distribution of the drug:

$$V_d = \frac{\text{dose}}{\text{blood concentration}}$$

17

The volume of distribution is not necessarily a true anatomical space. If it is five litres or less there is distribution into the blood compartment, while a volume of 5–20 litres implies that the drug is in the extracellular compartment, and one of about 40 litres implies it is distributed throughout body water. Some volumes of distribution are greater than total body water and this implies that the drug has been concentrated in one or other tissues.

Volume of distribution may be altered in critically ill patients for several reasons, such as altered protein binding, haemodilution, alterations in the distributions of body water, and treatment. Enthusiastic fluid administration, currently in vogue during resuscitation, may cause profound dilutional effects.[3]

Protein binding

Once a drug is in the blood it needs to be transported to the receptor or other site of action and to organs of elimination. Although there is information about transport within the blood, little is known about transport from the blood to the receptor, or the enzyme.

There are many proteins in the blood to which drugs may bind reversibly. These proteins are involved in the transport of drugs. Two are of special importance. The first, albumin, carries acidic drugs such as phenytoin and lignocaine; the other, α_1-acid glycoprotein, carries basic drugs such as morphine. Other proteins, such as lipoproteins, and erythrocytes also carry drugs.[4] Some drugs bind to more than one protein, for example prednisolone binds to both albumin and α_1-acid glycoprotein.

Protein binding markedly affects a drug's activity. Only the free, unbound drug diffuses easily to reach receptor sites and exert an effect. This free component is also the part that undergoes metabolism and elimination.

Drugs have a variable degree of protein binding. For example, ampicillin is 25% protein bound whereas cloxacillin is 90% protein bound. Some authors believe that highly protein-bound drugs are susceptible to displacement from their binding sites. For example, warfarin is 99% protein bound. If another drug which competes for its binding site, such as salicylate,[5] is given it may decrease the amount that is bound from 99% to 98%. Although this is a small change, the amount that is unbound and able to exert an effect, increases from 1% to 2%, a doubling. With warfarin this may result in overcoagulation. Other authors have contested the importance of displacement from binding sites, arguing that there is an instantaneous increase in drug elimination.[6] However, this may only occur in those drugs for which the liver enzymes are not saturated.

Albumin

Albumin carries many drugs. It has a molecular weight of about 68 000 Da and it is not surprising that there are variants of albumin. Several different types have been described, some with unimportant changes in their amino acid composition. The commonest, Albumin Lille, occurs with a frequency of 0·0006%. Interestingly, there are some humans who appear

18

to lack the genes to make significant amounts of albumin. Although small amounts are present, it is measured in mg/l rather than g/l.[7] These humans appear to be healthy apart from increased fat in their legs. Transport of hormones as well as drugs is thought to be another important function of albumin. However, in analbuminic rats, there does not appear to be any disturbance of thyroid stimulating hormone, which is transported by albumin. Albumin appears to have two binding sites. Drugs can be identified as binding to one or other site (Figure 2.1). The importance of amino acid changes on these is unknown.

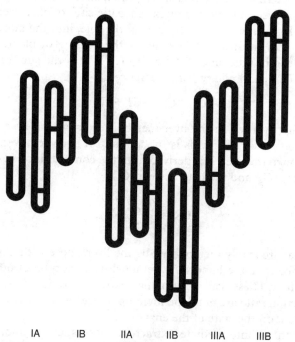

IA   IB   IIA   IIB   IIIA   IIIB

Figure 2.1   Schematic representation of the albumin molecule, showing several binding sites.

The mechanism of change and configuration has been described in pancreatitis. Kobayashi and colleagues[8] have shown that pancreatic enzymes may cause bisalbumin to appear. This is thought to be because albumin is secreted by the inflamed abdominal wall into the peritoneal cavity where the enzymes are partially digested. It is then absorbed into the circulation. Other changes in the electophoretic ability of albumin have been described in the critically ill.[9] These may be due to changes such as high-dose antibiotics, urea, or bilirubin.[8,10]

α_1-Acid glycoprotein

This protein increases after stress of many types, including surgery. Although it binds many drugs such as bupivacaine and might be expected

19

to decrease the free fraction of them, this has not been shown. There are several reasons for this. Like albumin, several different forms exist,[11] and it might also change with the severity and type of disease.[12] The concentration of α_1-acid glycoprotein increases in trauma,[13] surgery,[14] inflammation and chronic pain,[15] and carcinoma.[16]

Elimination

There are two components to elimination. The first is metabolism and the second, excretion. Metabolism is principally performed in the liver, although an increasing number of extrahepatic sites of drug metabolism is recognised. Excretion of most drugs is in the bile, into the gut or through the kidneys into the urine. Clearance is the volume of blood or plasma cleared of drug in unit time. Total clearance (Cl_t) is the sum of metabolic (Cl_m), renal (Cl_r), and biliary (Cl_b) clearances:

$$Cl_t = Cl_m + Cl_r + Cl_b$$

The avidity with which the liver metabolises drugs can be expressed as the extraction ratio (ER). This is the amount of drug removed during its passage through the liver. It is derived from the concentration of drug in the hepatic artery (C_a) and the hepatic vein (C_v):

$$ER = \frac{(C_a - C_v)}{C_a}$$

Drugs that are avidly metabolised by the liver, those with a high extraction ratio (for example lignocaine, fentanyl, and morphine) depend upon liver blood flow. These drugs have a high extraction ratio. Those drugs with a low extraction ratio are not dependent upon liver blood flow. Instead, they are dependent on the state of the enzyme.

Drugs with an intermediate extraction ratio, such as midazolam and alfentanil, are affected by changes in both. The elimination of most drugs occurs at a rate which is proportional to the concentration of the drug present, a constant fraction of the drug being eliminated in unit time. This is called first-order kinetics. However, if the enzyme system becomes saturated, then elimination proceeds at a constant rate. This is called zero-order kinetics. Ethanol and phenytoin have zero-order kinetics.

Half-life is the time taken for the plasma concentration of the drug to decrease by 50%. It is dependent upon the volume of distribution and clearance. The elimination half-life (t_{el}) is:

$$t_{el} = \frac{0.693 \times V_d}{Cl}$$

The kidneys are the most important organ involved in the excretion of drugs and their metabolites. Most drugs are lipid rather than water soluble and therefore need metabolising to become water soluble for excretion. The mechanisms involved in renal excretion include glomerular filtration, tubular secretion and reabsorption. Some drugs may undergo one of these mechanisms and others all of them. The molecular weight and charge of a molecule, the degree of protein binding, and the blood flow to the glomerulus all determine whether or not a drug can be filtered. Those substances that are eliminated by filtration are usually polar, unbound molecules, such as aminoglycosides.

In the proximal renal tubule, drugs (both acidic and basic) such as cimetidine and penicillin, are secreted by two different active transport mechanisms. Although only the unbound drug is able to cross membranes, this does not seem to hamper secretion. This is probably because the drugs rapidly dissociate from their binding proteins to maintain equilibrium. However, competition between substances for secretion may decrease the elimination of some drugs. For example, probenecid reduces the elimination of penicillin and prolongs its action. In the distal renal tubule, the passive reabsorption of weak acids occurs through the peritubular capillaries. This passive reabsorption depends on drugs being in the non-ionised, lipid-soluble form and is therefore influenced by urinary pH.

Acidic drugs (barbiturates and salicylates) are mostly non-ionised and lipid soluble in acid urine. They will, therefore, diffuse back across the distal renal tubule cell membranes and be reabsorbed and not excreted. To prevent reabsorption and enhance excretion of acidic drugs, the urine is made alkaline. This changes the drugs to an ionised polar form, which cannot cross cell membranes so increase excretion. The reverse may be applied for basic drugs.

In the critically ill, hypotension and drugs that reduce renal blood flow will lead to accumulation of drugs and metabolites excreted by the kidneys.

High molecular weight metabolites (4–500 Da) are excreted in the bile. Biliary excretion is usually less important than renal elimination for most drugs. In the liver, canalicular transport mechanisms transport ionised drug metabolites into the bile. This is an ATPase-dependent, saturable, non-specific process that can be inhibited by other drugs. This route of elimination in the critically ill has not been investigated and its importance is unknown.

Metabolism

The purpose of drug metabolism is to change an active, lipid-soluble compound into a water-soluble, inactive substance that can be excreted. Two phases are usually involved in this. The first phase, phase I metabolism, commonly involves cytochromes P450, although others enzymes also perform phase I metabolism including:

- alcohol dehydrogenase
- aldehyde dehydrogenase
- alkylhydrazine oxidase

- amine oxidases
- aromatases
- xanthine oxidase.

Phase I enzymes perform reactions such as oxidation and hydroxylation.

The metabolites produced by these enzymes may be less active, or highly active, or in some instances even toxic. Paracetamol (acetaminophen) is a frequently used analgesic. Most of the drug undergoes glucuronidation and sulphation, but a small amount is metabolised to a toxic metabolite (N-acetyl-p-benzoquinone [NAPQI]) by cytochrome P450 2E1. This toxic metabolite is inactivated by conjugation with glutathione. When large amounts of paracetamol have been ingested, glutathione supply becomes depleted and the toxic metabolite accumulates and can cause necrosis of the liver and poison the kidneys. The risk of hepatic damage is greater if the patient is taking an enzyme-inducing drug such as alcohol.

The phase I metabolite is usually metabolised further by a phase II enzyme. This enzyme conjugates the phase II metabolite with another group such as glutathione, a glucuronide, or a sulphide group. A drug that exemplifies these pathways is midazolam. It is metabolised by a cytochrome P450, first to 1-hydroxymidazolam and then to 1-hydroxymidazolam glucuronide.

A few drugs are metabolised mostly by phase II metabolism alone. Morphine is one such drug. It is metabolised to morphine-3-glucuronide (M3G) and morphine-6-glucuronide (M6G). When there are several pathways for the metabolism of one drug, there are many factors that influence by which pathway a drug is metabolised. Ismail and colleagues[17] studied this in rats infected with malaria and then given low and high doses of paracetamol. Overall, at low doses there was little change in the clearance of paracetamol. However, there was an increase in sulphation with an accompanying decrease in glucuronidation.[17] At high doses, sulphation was saturated and because of the reduction in glucuronidation, clearance reduced.

Enzymes

Cytochromes P450 are a family of haemoproteins. In humans, about 20 or so have been described. They are characterised by their amino acid homology. Families are identified by an Arabic number and have at least 40% amino acid homology. A sub-family is identified by a capital letter and has at least 55% amino acid homology. The gene product is identified by a further Arabic number.[18] This approach to nomenclature has replaced the older system of using substrate specificity and enzyme. Thus cytochrome P450 3A4 is nifedipine oxidase and cyclosporin oxidase.

Cytochromes P450 tend to be located predominantly in the central region of the hepatic lobule, whilst phase II enzymes tend to be distributed in the periportal region. Within the cell, cytochromes P450 are found on the endoplasmic reticulum and within the mitochondria. Phase II enzymes are located mostly in the cytoplasm.

There is a third group of enzymes that are becoming increasingly important for drug metabolism. These are the enzymes that are not present in large amounts in the liver, the so-called extrahepatic enzymes (most enzymes are found in low amounts outside the liver). Of these the most important are the blood and tissue esterases. One of them, butyrylcholinesterase (pseudocholinesterase), has been recognised for its importance in the metabolism of suxamethonium (succinylcholine). This muscle relaxant is completely broken down by butyrylcholinesterase. There are several genetic variants of this enzyme; some result in a prolonged effect. Many other drugs are now being designed to be metabolised either by butyrylcholinesterase or other esterases similar to it. Mivacurium, a non-depolarising neuromuscular blocking agent, is also metabolised by butyrylcholinesterase. However, despite being metabolised by other enzymes as well, it suffers the same difficulties in metabolism as suxamethonium.[19]

Remifentanil is an new opioid. It differs from the other opioids of the same group in that it is metabolised by many esterases. These enzymes are found in the blood and in the tissues. Because of the redundancy of the enzyme systems, this opioid is unlikely to be affected by the absence of one or even several of the esterases. This also makes remifentanil's metabolism independent of liver function. Studies during the anhepatic period of liver transplantation have shown its elimination to be normal.[20]

It is important to realise that each day the body has to metabolise many hundreds of xenobiotics (foreign substances) of which drugs are only one group. With the limited number of enzymes available to the body, most enzymes metabolise more than one substance.

Enzyme function may change because of inhibition or induction. Inhibition is usually quick while induction is slow. This is because enzyme induction results from an increased amount of enzyme, which takes time to occur.[21] Inhibition may occur after a single dose of a drug. It may be caused by direct interference with the enzyme itself, changes in the expression of the enzyme, or changes in the environment itself. Substrate inhibition may occur between midazolam and erythromycin, resulting in prolonged coma from the midazolam. Metabolite inhibition occurs with the antidepressant nortriptyline.[22] The phase I metabolite of nortriptyline inhibits the enzyme that produces it. Some drugs such as sulphinpyrazone can induce the metabolism of some drugs (for example, phenytoin and warfarin) and inhibit the metabolism of others (for example, theophylline). When drugs that induce or inhibit enzymes are withdrawn, the plasma concentration of the target drug may change, leading again to the possibility of treatment failure or toxicity if an adjustment to dose is not made.

Enzyme inhibition may at times be useful to prevent toxicity. Imipenem is an antibiotic broken down by the enzyme dehydropeptidase-1, found in the brush border microvilli of the proximal tubule. Inhibition of this enzyme by the addition of cilastatin delays the metabolism of imipenem, reducing the dose of the drug needed. It also means that active drug is present in the urine rather than inactive metabolites, allowing urinary infections to be treated.

There are many factors in the critically ill that may change drug metabolism. What it is important to realise is that drug metabolism is constantly changing as the patient's condition improves or worsens. Since phase I enzymes perform the first metabolic step, if they are changed, then all the steps in the metabolism of the drug will be affected. Cytochromes P450 are present in smaller amounts than phase II enzymes. Furthermore, they are more sensitive to disease and its effects than phase II enzymes. The understanding of these enzymes is therefore crucial to an understanding of drug metabolism and the next section will concentrate on these enzymes. There are many factors that contribute to changing enzyme function including the following:

Systemic inflammatory response syndrome (SIRS)

This term is used in an attempt to define non-specific inflammation in the body resulting from many causes including infection, pancreatitis, etc.[23] SIRS affects most of the body rather than a single organ and inflammation is the essential part. Since infection is but one cause, a positive microbiological culture is not an essential part of the syndrome.

Many inflammatory mediators are released in sepsis, including interleukins (IL) 1, 4, and 6, tumour necrosis factor and interferon (IFN-γ).[9] The release of any of these can be triggered by endotoxin itself, an important course of changes in drug metabolism.[24-28]

In animals, endotoxin has been shown to reduce the amount of cytochromes P450 and its activity.[24,26] These changes are associated with a reduction in mRNA.[26] Interleukin-1 has also been shown to produce similar changes.[28] Information from humans is limited and most results are from studies in hepatocytes grown in primary culture. We have shown that serum from critically ill humans contains a substance that appears to inhibit the enzymes as well. Others have shown that individual cytokines affect the hepatic expressions of cytochromes P450 differently (Table 2.1).

In a further study with serum from critically ill patients in which we incubated microsomes with serum from critically ill patients, we showed there was significant inhibition of the metabolism of midazolam.[30] The substance

Table 2.1 The effect of inflammatory mediators on various drug metabolising enzymes.[29] ↓ = decrease, ↑ = increase, ⟷ = unchanged

Cytochrome P450 (CYP)	IL-1β	IL-4	IL-6	TNF-α	IFN-γ
CYP 1A2	↓	↓	↓	↓	↓
CYP 2C	↓	↓	↓	↓	⟷
CYP 2E1	↓	↑5x	↓	↓	↓
CYP 3A	↓	⟷	↓	↓	⟷
Epoxide hydrolase	↓	No data	↓	↓	⟷

that caused this was unknown. However, some workers have suggested that propofol may be an enzyme inhibitor. Some of the patients from which we took serum had received propofol. In a later study we showed that propofol is not an enzyme inhibitor at clinical concentrations.[31]

Viral illness is also known to depress drug metabolism[32] and interferon is a probable cause. Interferon[33-35] may exert its effect in three ways. There may be release of a secondary mediator such as IL-1. Alternatively, interferon may induce xanthine oxidase which increases the amount of free radicals present and may interfere with normal cell functions. Finally, interferon may enhance haem turnover, reducing the amount of cytochromes P450 present.[36]

Hypoxia

In the critically ill cellular hypoxia is common. In the liver this may be because of a reduction of liver blood flow. Oxygen is an important substrate and energy source for drug metabolism. Not all enzymes are equally affected by hypoxia, as oxidation reactions appear to be more sensitive to hypoxia than sulphation.

Oxygen is needed by the hepatocytes to metabolise drugs for several reasons:

- to produce energy for metabolism
- as a substrate for drug oxidation
- as a terminal electron acceptor
- for processors dependent on oxidation equilibrium (redox potential of the cell)

Hypoxia has been shown to reduce cytochrome P450 3A4 expression in human hepatocytes in primary culture.[37] Most studies in intact animals have been performed in those made chronically hypoxic. This is because the compensatory cardiorespiratory changes associated with acute hypoxia make it difficult to study the effects of hypoxia. Drugs which increase oxygen consumption may also exacerbate the changes in drug metabolism caused by hypoxia and lead to ischaemic hepatitis.[38] Many drugs used in the critically ill increase oxygen consumption and this can be prevented by a cytochrome P450 inhibitor.[39]

The liver is particularly sensitive to hypoxia because 70% of its blood supply is from the portal vein, which has blood with low oxygen content. The remaining 30% is from the hepatic artery with a high oxygen content. This dual supply leads to large differences in oxygen supply to different parts of the liver. Those near to the artery have a good oxygen supply, whereas those further removed do not. These hepatocytes are particularly sensitive to systemic hypoxia and poor blood flow because their oxygen supply is so critical.

In rats the lowest fractional oxygen concentration inspired oxygen (F_{IO_2}) allowing survival is 0·07. However, liver damage occurs at this concentration. At an F_{IO_2} lower than this the rats start to die and liver damage in the

25

survivors is greater. Isolated hepatocytes survive in oxygen tensions as low as 0·1 mmHg. However, they do not function normally[40] and an oxygen tension of 2–10 mmHg (3–14 μmol/l is needed for energy production.

A German group[41] measured the amount of cytochrome P450 from a needle biopsy in patients dying with and without shock after myocardial infarction. In addition, they measured the steady state plasma concentration of lignocaine after an infusion. Patients with shock had a reduced clearance and higher plasma concentration of lignocaine. When given dobutamine to increase cardiac output, the plasma concentrations of lignocaine decreased.

The time taken for hypoxia to induce changes in drug metabolising enzymes is short. Rabbits exposed to a low F_{IO_2} reduced their ability to metabolise theophylline within 8 hours.[42]

Temperature

Fever is common in the critically ill. Although increasing the temperature usually increases the rate of a chemical reaction, this is not always so with drug metabolism. In volunteers who had a fever induced with a pyrogen, antipyrine, metabolism was reduced.[33] Similarly, quinine metabolism is also reduced during acute malaria and steroid-induced fever.[43] These findings may be explained by the cause of the fever. Both the injection of a pyrogen and an acute illness cause the release of inflammatory mediators and these will reduce the expression and function of enzymes.

Hypothermia has been investigated during cardiopulmonary bypass. Patients were given esmolol by continuous infusion; as the patient was cooled, plasma concentrations of esmolol increased, showing a reduction in clearance because of a reduction in its metabolism.[44] This model of temperature change does not involve the release of inflammatory mediators and this may explain the differences between studies looking at fever and this one.

Nutrition

Critically ill patients do not have a normal diet. A change in diet, deficiencies, or excesses of a variety of dietary components is associated with abnormal enzyme function.[45-52] Starvation and malnutrition cause further changes,[48,50,52] in particular an increase in cytochrome P450 2E1.[45] Interestingly, this change may be blocked by the sedative chlormethiazole.[53] Similarly, vitamin C deficiency in guinea pigs is associated with a decrease in cytochromes P450.[46] Although scurvy is rare, lack of other vitamins and trace elements, which may occur in the critically ill, may result in similar changes. High-protein, high-lipid or low-carbohydrate diets all lead to an increase in cytochrome P450,[51] and an increase in clearance drugs such as theophylline. High-fat diets when given as part of parenteral nutrition increase the oxidation of antipyrine.[54] The fat is thought to stimulate the growth hormone, which in turn changes gene subscription, resulting in an increase in cytochrome P450 2E1.

26

Stress

Patients in the ICU are stressed. Not only is there the physical stress of being critically ill, but the environment itself is also stressful. Pollack and colleagues studied non-traumatic stress in rats.[55] He exposed animals to flashing lights, rocking cages, food and water deprivation, and finally made the rats swim in cold water. After this they measured antipyrine clearance to look at enzyme function. They found it was reduced in the stressed compared with the unstressed animals. They also measured indocyanine green clearance as a marker of liver blood flow. Again, in the stressed animals this was reduced, showing a reduction in liver blood flow. One of several possible mechanisms for the effect of stress on antipyrine clearance is that the stress released catecholamines. These in turn reduced liver blood flow, making the hepatocytes more hypoxic, so reducing enzyme expression with its consequent results on antipyrine clearance.

Age

There are many changes that accompany ageing, including a reduction in cardiac output, body weight, body water, plasma and albumin concentration, and an increase in body fat. There are also significant changes in the elderly in the elimination half-life and clearance of drugs metabolised by cytochromes P450 (Table 2.2). The mechanisms behind these changes are unknown.

Phase II enzymes also change. Morphine metabolism has been studied in premature infants. Choonara *et al.*[56] showed that the clearance of morphine was decreased compared with term infants. Metabolite patterns were also different. The M3G:morphine ratio in plasma and urine and M6G:morphine ratio in urine were higher in children than neonates. This shows that there is enhancement of glucuronidation pathways with growth. Since there was no difference in the M3G:M6G ratio in neonates compared with that in children, the metabolic pathways develop together.

Table 2.2   Effects of ageing in humans on various pharmacokinetic variables of drugs metabolised by cytochromes P450 (from[57]).

Drug	Age (years)	Plasma half-life $(t_{1/2})$ (h)	Plasma clearance (ml/kg/h)
Aminopyrine	25–30	3	
	65–85	10	
Antipyrine	20–40	12·5	
	65–92	16·8	
Phenobarbitone	20–40	71	
	50–60	77	
	70	107	
Phenytoin	20–43		26
	67–95		42

Sex

In some animals there is a marked sex difference. In rats the injections of endotoxin leads to a more rapid decrease and recovery in cytochromes P450 and their mRNA in females.[26] Whether this occurs in humans is unknown. However, we and others have shown a different expression in cytochrome P450 3A4 between males and females.[58]

Endocrine disorders

Endocrine disease is probably more common in the critically ill than is recognised. The disease the patient presents with, or the treatment, may cause it, or alternatively the patient may have it chronically.

Liver and renal failure

This subject is discussed in detail in Chapters 4 and 5. However, a brief overview is given here for completeness. Liver and renal failure will both change enzyme expression and function. Acute fulminant liver failure will remove the metabolic ability of the liver to a variable degree. This will depend on the severity of the liver failure. Although we have shown in several studies that there is significant extrahepatic metabolism of drugs,[59-62] most metabolism still occurs in the liver. Also, it should be noted that any process that affects the liver, causing liver failure, will almost certainly affect the enzymes found at extrahepatic sites to a variable degree. Chronic liver disease also affects drug metabolism. It may do so in one of two ways. In cirrhotic livers enzyme expression may be normal, but the architecture of the liver is distorted. This results in a variable blood flow to hepatocytes, reducing delivery of the drug to them. In other conditions associated with hepatocellular damage, blood flow is normal but enzyme function is reduced.

Renal failure also changes drug metabolism both experimentally and in humans.[63-65] After bilateral subtotal nephrectomy in rats there is a decrease in hepatic cytochromes P450.[64] However, the change in cytochrome P450 function varies between drugs. For example propranolol is eliminated poorly in liver failure[66] whilst the elimination of phenytoin is increased in uraemic patients.[67]

Pharmacogenetics

There is considerable interpatient variability in the effects of drugs. Although most of this is due to the patient's phenotype, in some instances it may be owing to genotype. One of the best studied pharmacogenetic abnormalities is the metabolism of suxamethonium; there are four major genotypes based on substrate metabolism. They are usually silent, atypical to fluoride resistance. If the patient is homozygous for the atypical and silent form and given suxamethonium, prolonged apnoea will result.

Cytochrome P450 2D6 is another enzyme that is affected by genetic polymorphism and several forms have been identified.[68] The first descriptions of an abnormality with this enzyme were with the antihypertensive drug debrisoquine. However, this enzyme metabolises many other drugs including β-blockers, morphine, and codeine. Since codeine is metabolised by cytochrome P450 2D6 to morphine and then exerts its effects and 10% of the population do not posses this enzyme, this may go some way to explain the ineffective analgesia some patients get with codeine.

Metabolites

There is increasing recognition of the activity of the metabolites of drugs in the critically ill. This may range from toxicity (see paracetamol above) to prolongation of clinical effects. In the sedative and analgesic group of drugs, morphine has long been recognised as having active metabolites. Morphine-6-glucuronide (M6G) is thought to have an activity 40 times the parent drug for sedation and analgesia. Some authors believe that morphine-3 glucuronide (M3G) antagonises this.[69,70] The balance of the two metabolites may determine how much analgesia a patient gets. Both M3G and M6G are polar substances that are excreted in the kidney. Polar substances cannot cross membranes and so have pharmacological activity. Carrupt and colleagues[71] have shown that M3G and M6G can change their configuration, affecting their solubility. Thus in a lipid environment these metabolites are fat soluble and in an aqueous environment they are water soluble. Midazolam also has a glucuronide that is active. Unlike morphine, its activity is only one-fortieth of the activity of the parent drug. Similarly, the new opioid remifentanil has an active metabolite, but this is only

Table 2.3 Important metabolites of sedative and analgesic drugs (reproduced from[72]).

Parent drug	Metabolite	Comments
Diazepam	Nordesmethyl diazepam, oxazepam	Both of these are active sedatives. They have a longer elimination half-life than diazepam. The elimination half-life of nordesmethyl diazepam can increase to 403 h
Midazolam	l-Hydroxymidazolam	10% of the activity of the parent drug
Midazolam	l-Hydroxymidazolam glucuronide	Accumulates in renal failure and has one-quarter the activity of midazolam
Morphine	Morphine-3-glucuronide	Antianalgesic
	Morphine-6-glucuronide	Potent analgesic properties, up to 40 times more active than parent drug when given intracisternly. Longer duration of action than morphine. Will be retained in renal failure
Vecuronium	Nordesacetyl vecuronium	Activity enhanced by hypomagnesaemia
Pethidine	Norpethidine	Can cause fits

29

one-four thousandth the activity of the parent drug. It is interesting to note that as newer drugs are being developed, attention is being paid to their metabolite and these are becoming far less active. Other drugs with active metabolites are shown in Table 2.3.

Drug reactions and interactions

Drug reactions and interactions are numerous and range from mild non-threatening rashes to fatal anaphylaxis.

There are several ways that there may be reactions to drugs. The reaction may be predictable, such as a recognised side effect of toxicity, or known drug interaction. The example given above of erythromycin inhibiting the enzyme responsible for the metabolism of midazolam is one of these. Prolonged coma is the result of this interaction.[73-75] Unpredictable reactions include previously unknown drug interactions, allergy, and idiosyncratic reactions. Also included is intolerance, which is an exaggerated pharmacological or toxic effect of the drug.

Some adverse reactions may be errors due to mistakes in drug delivery. In a paediatric intensive care unit Bordun and Butt[76] found errors in drug prescription, administration, and drug interactions in 2% of prescriptions. Of these errors, 12% resulted in harm to the patient. A further study of adverse drug reactions, also in a paediatric intensive care unit, showed 76 adverse reactions in 899 patients. The most commonly involved drugs were midazolam, morphine, salbutamol, vecuronium, hydrocortisone, and theophylline. These reactions mostly occurred when drugs were being used outside the product license.[77]

Many adverse drug reactions go unrecognised in the critically ill patient because the signs and symptoms may be masked or may be attributable to the illness or another drug and patients are unable to complain of symptoms.

Idiosyncratic reactions are a mixed group, which are not predictable from the pharmacological action of the drug. Some of them may be caused by pharmacogenetic alterations.

An interesting adverse effect is vancomycin and the red man syndrome. The increase in methicillin-resistant *Staphylococcus aureus* has increased the use of vancomycin in intensive care units. If it is given quickly, the red man syndrome, characterised by flushing, pruritis, angio-oedema, and occasionally cardiovascular depression, may be seen. This is caused by histamine release which frequently occurs when doses of 1000 mg are given by infusion. It is worse with the first dose and related to the rate of infusion. When Polk *et al.* studied 11 volunteers, they found that 9 experienced some aspect of the syndrome and 4 had a severe reaction.[78] Not all drug interactions are harmful. Synergistic combinations of drugs may lead to an improved therapeutic effect, with a reduction of dose and adverse effects. It has been widely used in other areas of medicine. Combinations of induction agents during anaesthesia[79-81] is one area that is being applied to the critically ill.

Reducing adverse effects is another area. Imipenem was found to be nephrotoxic in animals. However, it was not the imipenem that was nephrotoxic, but a metabolite. The enzyme dehydropeptidase-1, found in the proximal renal tubular cells, produced this metabolite by inactivating imipenem by hydrolysing its β-lactam ring.[82]

Multiple drug interactions may also occur in the critically ill because of the number of drugs they are given. Zylber-Katz has reported such a patient, receiving cyclosporin, rifampicin, isoniazid, and erythromycin. The plasma concentration of cyclosporin was low at first, thought to be caused by the induction of CYP 3A4 by rifampicin. When the rifampicin and isoniazid was stopped, the concentration of cyclosporin increased to toxic concentrations because the erythromycin acted as an enzyme inhibitor, prolonging the elimination of cyclosporin.[83]

Effects on multiple organ systems

Although a drug is usually given to target a single organ, often they have effects elsewhere. Morphine, for example, is given for analgesia, but as discussed above, it may have effects on drug metabolism mediated through growth hormone.[84]

Opioids may also play a part in immune suppression. Several studies have looked at the effects of opioids on white cell function (Table 2.4). All seem to show a depression of this after opioids; however, the importance of this in the critically ill still needs to be shown.

Similarly, catecholamines are given to change the function of the cardiovascular system. It now appears that they may also have significant effects in the endocrine system and also white cell function.[85,86]

Table 2.4   The effects of opioids on white cell function.

Study	Opioid	Subject	Effect
Tubaro et al. (1983)[87]	Morphine	Mice	↓ Phagocytosis ↓ Killing
Moudgil et al. (1981)[88]	Morphine Diazepam IV induction	Leucocytes	↓ Phagocytosis
Edwards et al. (1984)[89]	Anaesthesia	Humans	↓ Migration
Yeager et al. (1995)[90]	Morphine	Volunteers	↓ Killer cell activity

Conclusion

The way in which a drug behaves in the critically ill cannot be reliably predicted. Its effects will change as the condition of the patient alters. An understanding of the pharmacodynamic and pharmacokinetic principles will help in understanding basic drug actions. It is essential to constantly

31

review the effect a drug has on the critically ill and act on it accordingly. When caring for a critically ill patient and thinking about drugs one should ask:

- Is the drug really needed?
- Is the drug doing what I want?
- Do the benefits outweigh the risk?
- Can another safer drug be used instead?
- When can the drug be stopped?

and in these days of financial constraint and health care systems:

- Can an equally good and equally safe but cheaper drug be used instead?

1 Kong KL, Willatts SM, Prys-Roberts C. Isoflurane compared with midazolam for sedation in the intensive care unit. *BMJ* 1989;**298**:1277-9.
2 Spencer EM, Willatts SM. Isoflurane for prolonged sedation in the intensive care unit;efficacy and safety. *Intens Care Med* 1992;**18**:415-21.
3 Van Heerden PV, Chew G. Severe hypokalaemia due to lignocaine toxicity. *Anaesth Intens Care* 1996;**24**:128-9.
4 Bickel MH. Binding of chlorpromazine and imipramine to red cells, albumin, lipoproteins, and other blood components. *J Pharm Pharmacol* 1975;**27**:733-8.
5 Wood M. Plasma drug binding: implications for anesthesiologists. *Anesth Analg* 1986;**65**:786-804.
6 Rolan PE. Plasma protein binding displacement interactions – why are they still regarded as clinically important? *Br J Clin Pharmacol* 1994;**37**:125-8.
7 McKusick VA, Francomano CA, Antonarakis SE. Autosomal dominant phenotypes. In: *Mendelian inheritance in man*. Baltimore and London: Johns Hopkins University Press. 1991;39-44.
8 Kobayashi S, Okamura N, Kamoi K, Sugita O. Bisalbumin (fast and slow type) induced by human pancreatic juice. *Ann Clin Biochem* 1995;**32**:63-7.
9 Park GR. Molecular mechanisms of drug metabolism in the critically ill. *Br J Anaesth* 1996;**77**:32-49.
10 Lapresle C, Wal J-M. The binding of penicillin to albumin molecules in bisalbuminemia induced by penicillin therapy. *Biochim Biophys Acta* 1979;**586**:106-11.
11 Serbource-Goguel N, Corbic M, Erlinger S, Durand G, Agnerey J, Feger J. Measurement of serum 1-acid glycoprotein and 1-antitrypsin desialylation in liver disease. *Hepatology* 1983;**3**:356-9.
12 Mackiewicz A, Khan MA, Gorny A *et al.* Glycoforms of alphal-acid glycoprotein in sera of human immunodeficiency virus-infected patients. *J Infect Dis* 1994;**169**:1360-3.
13 Edwards DJ, Lalka D, Cerra F, Slaughter RL. Alpha$_1$-acid glycoprotein concentration and protein binding in trauma. *Clin Pharmacol Ther* 1982;**31**:62-7.
14 Fremstad D, Bergerud K, Haffner JFW, Lunde PKM. Increased plasma binding of quinidine after surgery:a preliminary report. *Eur J Clin Pharmacol* 1976;**10**:441-4.
15 Fukui T, Hameroff SR, Gandolfi AJ. Alpha$_1$-acid glycoprotein and beta-endorphin alterations in chronic pain patients. *Anesthesiology* 1984;**60**:494-6.
16 Tatman AJ, Wrigley SR, Jones RM. Resistance to atracurium in a patient with an increase in plasma alpha$_1$-globulins. *Br J Anaesth* 1991;**67**:623-5.
17 Ismail S, Kokwaro GO, Back DJ, Edwards G. Effect of malaria infection on pharmacokinetics of paracetamol in rat. *Xenobiotica* 1994;**24**:527-33.
18 Nebert DW, Nelson DR, Coon MJ *et al.* The P450 superfamily:update on new sequences, gene mapping, and recommended nomenclature. *DNA Cell Biol* 1991;**10**:1-14.
19 Ostengaard D, Jensen FS, Jensen E, Skovgaard LT, Viby-Mogensen J. Mivacurium-induced neuromuscular blockade in patients with atypical plasma cholinesterase. *Acta Anaesthesiol Scand* 1993;**37**:314-18.
20 Navapurkar V, Archer S, Gupta SK, Frazer N, Muir SK, Park GR. Pharmacokinetics of remifentanil during hepatic transplantation. *Br J Anaesth* 1998;**81**:881-6.
21 Barry M, Feely J. Enzyme induction and inhibition. *Pharmacol Ther* 1990;**48**:71-94.

22 Murray M. Metabolite intermediate complexation of microsomal cytochrome P450 2C11 in male rat liver by nortriptyline. *Mol Pharmacol* 1992;**42**:931–8.

23 Bone RC, Balk RA, Cerra FB *et al*. Definitions for sepsis and organ failure and guidelines for the use on innovative therapies in sepsis. *Chest* 1992;**101**:1644–55.

24 Egawa K, Yoshida M, Kasai N. An endotoxin-induced serum factor that depresses hepatic δ-aminolevulinic acid synthetase activity and cytochrome P-450 levels in mice. *Microbiol Immunol* 1981;**25**:1091–6.

25 Ghezzi P, Saccardo B, Villa P, Rossi V, Bianchi M, Dinarrelo CA. Role of interleukin-1 in the depression of liver drug metabolism by endotoxin. *Infect Immun* 1986;**54**:837–40.

26 Morgan ET. Suppression of constitutive cytochrome P450 gene expression in livers of rats undergoing an acute phase response to endotoxin. *Mol Pharmacol* 1989;**36**:699–707.

27 Schaefer CF, Biber B, Lerner MR, Jöbsis-Vander Vliet FF, Fagraeus L. Rapid reduction of intestinal cytochrome a,a_3 during lethal endotoxemia. *J Surg Res* 1991;**51**:382–91.

28 Shedlofsky SI, Swim AT, Robinson JM, Gallicchio VS, Cohen DA, McClain CJ. Interleukin-1 (IL1) depresses cytochrome P450 levels and activity in mice. *Life Sci* 1987;**40**:2331–6.

29 Abdel-Razzak Z, Loyer P, Fautrel A *et al*. Cytokines down-regulate expression of major cytochrome P-450 enzymes in adult human hepatocytes in primary culture. *Mol Pharmacol* 1993;**44**:707–15.

30 Park GR, Miller E, Navapurkar V. What changes drug metabolism in critically ill patients? II Serum inhibits the metabolism of midazolam in human microsomes. *Anaesthesia* 1996;**51**:11–15.

31 Leung BP, Miller E, Park GR. The effect of propofol on midazolam metabolism in human liver microsome suspension. *Anaesthesia* 1997;**52**:945–8.

32 Chang KC, Laner BA, Bell JD, Chai H. Altered theophylline pharmacokinetics during acute respiratory viral illness. *Lancet* 1978;**1**:1132–3.

33 Elin RJ, Vesell ES, Wolff SM. Effects of etiocholanolone induced fever on plasma antipyrine half lives and metabolic clearance. *Clin Pharmacol Ther* 1975;**17**:447–57.

34 Moochhala SM. Alteration of drug biotransformation by interferon and host defense mechanism. *Ann Acad Med* 1991;**20**:13–18.

35 Morgan ET, Norman CA. Pretranslational suppression of cytochrome P-450h (IIC1l) gene expression in rat liver after administration of interferon inducers. *Drug Metab Dispos* 1990;**18**:649–53.

36 Ghezzi P, Saccardo B, Bianchi M. Induction of xanthine oxidase and heme oxygenase and depression of liver drug metabolism by interferon:a study with different recombinant interferons. *J Interferon Res* 1986;**6**:251–6.

37 Park GR, Pichard L, Tinel M *et al*. What changes drug metabolism in critically ill patients? Two preliminary studies in isolated hepatocytes. *Anaesthesia* 1994;**49**:188–91.

38 Gibson PR, Dudley FJ. Ischemic hepatitis: clinical features, diagnosis and prognosis. *Aust N Z J Med* 1984;**14**:822–5.

39 Becker GL. Effects of nonvolatile agents on oxygen demand and energy status in isolated hepatocytes. *Anesth Analg* 1988;**67**:923–8.

40 Anundi I, de Groot H. Hypoxic liver cell death:critical Po_2 and dependence of viability on glycolysis. *Am J Physiol* 1989;**257**:G58–64.

41 Gallenkamp H, Epping J, Fuchshofen-Rockel M, Heusler H, Richter E. Zytochrom P 450-gehalt und Arzneimittelmetabolismus der Leber im Schock. *Verh Dtsch Ges Inn Med* 1982;**88**:1093–6.

42 Du Souich P, Corteau H, Kobusch AB, Dalkara S, Ong H. Effect of hypoxia on the cytochrome P450 and theophylline metabolism. *Eur J Pharmacol* 1990;**183**:2122–3.

43 Trenholme GM, Williams RL, Rieckmann KH, Frischer H, Carson PE. Quinine disposition during malaria and during induced fever. *Clin Pharmacol Ther* 1976;**19**:459–67.

44 Jacobs JR, Croughwell ND, Goodman DK, White WD, Reves JG. Effect of hypothermia and sampling site on blood esmolol concentrations. *J Clin Pharmacol* 1993;**33**:360–5.

45 Johansson I, Lindros KO, Erikasson H, Ingelman-Sundberg M. Transcriptional control of CYP 2E1 in the perivenous liver region and during starvation. *Biochem Biophys Res Commun* 1990;**173**:331–8.

46 Kanazawa Y, Kitada M, Mori T. Ascorbic acid deficiency decreases specific forms of cytochrome P-450 in liver microsomes of guinea pigs. *Mol Pharmacol* 1991;**39**:456–60.

47 Kappas A, Anderson KE, Conney AH, Alvares AP. Influence of dietary protein and carbohydrate on antipyrine and theophylline metabolism in man. *Clin Pharmacol Ther* 1976;**20**:643–53.

48 Krishnaswamy K, Naidu AD. Microsomal enzymes in malnutrition as determined by plasma half-life of antipyrine. *BMJ* 1977;**1**:538–40.
49 Pineau T, Daujat M, Pichard L *et al*. Developmental expression of rabbit cytochrome P450 CYP1A1, CYP1A2 and CYP3A6 genes. Effect of weaning and rifampacin. *Eur J Biochem* 1991;**197**:145–53.
50 Shobha JC, Raghuram TC, Deva Kumar A, Krishnaswamy K. Antipyrine kinetics in undernourished diabetics. *Eur J Clin Pharmacol* 1991;**41**:359–61.
51 Yang CS, Brady JF, Hong J. Dietary effects on cytochrome P450, xenobiotic metabolism and toxicity. *FASEB* 1992;**6**:737–44.
52 Hu Y, Mishin V, Johansson I *et al*. Chlormethiazole as an efficient inhibitor of cytochrome P450 2E1 expression in rat liver. *J Pharmacol Exp Ther* 1994;**269**:1286–91.
53 Miahin V, von Bahr C, Ingelman-Sundberg M. Chlormethiazole as a potent and selective inhibitor in vivo of CYP2E1 during food deprivation. Abstract presented at the First International Conferance on Food Nutrition and Chemical Toxicity, Guildford, England, 1991.
54 Burgess P, Hall RI, Bateman DN, Johnston IDA. The effect of total parenteral nutrition on hepatic drug oxidation. *J Parenter Enteral Nutr* 1987;**11**:540–3.
55 Pollack GM, Browne JL, Marton J, Haberer LJ. Chronic stress impairs oxidative metabolism and hepatic excretion of model xenobiotic substrates in the rat. *Drug Metab Disp* 1991;**19**:130–4.
56 Choonara IA, McKay P, Hain R, Rane A. Morphine metabolism in children. *Br J Clin Pharmacol* 1989;**28**:599–604.
57 Schumucker DL. Drug deposition in the elderly: a review of the critical factors. *J Am Geriatr Soc* 1984;**32**:144–9.
58 Tarbit MH, Bayliss MK, Herriott D *et al*. Applications of molecular biology and in vitro technology to drug metabolism studies: an industrial perspective. *Biochem Soc Trans* 1993;**21**:1018–23.
59 Bodenham A, Quinn K, Park GR. Extra-hepatic metabolism of morphine. *Br J Anaesth* 1989;**63**:380–4.
60 Gray P, Park GR, Cockshott ID, Douglas ED, Shuker B, Simons PJ. Propofol metabolism in man during the anhepatic and reperfusion phases of liver transplantation. *Xenobiotica* 1992;**22**:105–14.
61 Gray P, Park GR. Plasma concentrations of dopexamine during the anhepatic period of liver transplantation. *Br J Clin Pharmacol* 1993;**37**:92.
62 Park GR, Manara AR, Dawling S. Extrahepatic metabolism of midazolam. *Br J Clin Pharmacol* 1989;**27**:634–7.
63 Elston A, Bayliss MK, Park GR. Effect of renal failure on drug metabolism by the liver. *Br J Anaesth* 1993;**71**:282–90.
64 Farrell GC. Drug metabolism in extrahepatic disease. *Pharmacol Ther* 1987;**35**:375–404.
65 Reidenberg MM. The biotranformations of drugs in renal failure. *Am J Med* 1977;**62**: 482–5.
66 Bianchetti G, Graziani G, Branicaccio D. Pharmacokinetics and effects of propanolol in terminal uraemic patients and in patients undergoing regular dialysis treatment. *Clin Pharmacokin* 1976;**1**:373–84.
67 Odar-Cederlof I, Borga O. Kinetics of diphenylhydantoin in uremic patients: consequences of decreased plasma protein binding. *Eur J Clin Pharmacol* 1974;**7**:31–7.
68 Idle J. Enigmatic variations. *Nature* 1988;**331**:391–2.
69 Gong QL, Hedner J, Bjorkman R, Hedner T. Morphine-3-glucuronide may functionally antagonize morphine-6-glucuronide induced antinociception and ventilatory depression in the rat. *Pain* 1992;**48**:249–55.
70 Smith MT, Watt JA, Cramond T. Morphine-3-glucuronide a potent antagonist of morphine analgesia. *Life Sci* 1990;**47**:579–85.
71 Carrupt PA, Testa B, Bechalany A, El Tayar N, Descas P, Perrissoud D. Morphine 6-glucuronide and morphine 3-glucuronide as molecular chameleons with unexpected lipophilicity. *J Med Chem* 1991;**34**:1272–5.
72 Park GR, Navapurkar VU, Koller J. Pharmacology of sedative and analgesic agents in the critically ill. In: Park GR, Sladen RN, eds. *Sedation and analgesia in the critically ill*. Oxford:Blackwell Science, 1995;18–50.
73 Hiller A, Olkkola KT, Isohanni P, Saarnivaara L. Unconsciousness associated with midazolam and erythromycin. *Br J Anaesth* 1990;**65**:826–8.
74 Olkkola KT, Aranko K, Luurila H *et al*. A potentially hazardous interaction between erythromycin and midazolam. *Clin Pharmacol Ther* 1993;**53**:298–305.

34

75 Wood M. Midazolam and erythromycin. *Br J Anaesth* 1991;**67**:131.
76 Bordun LA, Butt W. Drug errors in intensive care. *J Paediatr Child Health* 1992;**28**:309–11.
77 Gill AM, Leach HJ, Hughes J, Barker C, Nunn AJ, Choonara I. Adverse drug reactions in a paediatric intensive care unit. *Acta Paediatr* 1995;**84**(4):438–41.
78 Polk RE, Healy DP, Schwartz LB, Rock DT, Garson ML, Roller K. Vancomycin and the red man syndrome: pharmacodynamics of histamin release. *J Infect Dis* 1988;**157**(3): 502–7.
79 Short TG, Chui PT. Propofol and midazolam act synergistically in combination. *Br J Anaesth* 1991;**67**:539–45.
80 Park GR. Cosedation during spinal anaesthesia. *Anaesthesia* 1996;**51**:706–7.
81 Park GR, Godsiff L, Magee L. Cosedation in the critically ill. *Anaesthesia* 1995;**50**:1004–5.
82 Favero AD. Clinically important aspects of carbapenem safety. *Curr Opin Infect Dis* 1994;**7**:S38–42.
83 Zylber-Katz E. Multiple drug interactions with cyclosporine in a heart transplant patient. *Ann Pharmacother* 1995;**29**(2):127–31.
84 Rane A, Liu Z, Henderson CJ, Wolf CR. Divergent regulation of cytochrome P450 enzymes by morphine and pethidine; a neuroendocrine mechanism? *Mol Pharmacol* 1995;**47**:57–64.
85 Park GR, Couzens S, Hoskins RD. Effects of inotropes on platelet numbers and function. *Clin Intens Care* 1992;**3**:160–5.
86 Burns A, Brown D, Park GR. The effect of inotropes on leucocyte numbers, neutrophil function and lymphocyte subtypes. *Br J Anaesth* 1997;**78**:530–5.
87 Tubaro E, Borelli G, Croce C, Cavallo G, Santiangeli C. Effect of morphine on resistance to infection. *J Infect Dis* 1983;**148**:656–66.
88 Moudgil GC, Forrest JB, Gordon J. Comparative effects of volatile anaesthetics and nitrous oxide on human leukocyte chemotaxis in vitro. *Can J Anaesth* 1984;**31**:631–7.
89 Edwards AE, Gemmel LW, Mankin PP, Smith CJ, Allen JC, Hunter A. The effect of three differing anaesthetics on immune response. *Anaesthesia* 1984;**39**:1071–8.
90 Yeager MP, Colacchio TA, Yu CT. Morphine inhibits spontaneous and cytokine enhanced natural killer cell cytotoxicity in volunteers. *Anesthesiology* 1995;**83**:500–8.

3: Drug action

BARBARA J PLEUVRY

The study of mechanisms by which drugs can modify cellular and ultimately whole animal performance is still one of the most exciting and useful branches of science. It encompasses all branches of biological research such as molecular biology, cellular biology, microbiology, immunology, and genetics, as well physiology and pathology. It is a continuing hope that our increasing understanding of the molecular changes involved in body function will yield therapeutic breakthroughs in the years to come. It is also important not to lose sight of the fact that any drug must act in the whole body and these effects may not be predictable from known molecular interactions. An example is the application of gene therapy to the treatment of cystic fibrosis where the major problem affecting success of therapy was penetration of the delivery system to the appropriate cells.[1]

Mechanisms of drug action

While some drugs such as the osmotic diuretics and antacids do not bind to any particular cellular component in order to produce their effects, this mechanism of action is the exception, rather than the rule. Most drugs bind to proteins, although some antitumour and antimicrobial drugs may target DNA. Traditionally, general anaesthetics have been thought to interact with membrane lipids but this has been questioned as more is revealed about how general anaesthetics change modulation of neurotransmitter receptors, such as $GABA_A$[2] and $5HT_3$.[3] Indeed, the most sensitive receptors to general anaesthetic modulation are all genetically related pentameric receptors known as the ligand-gated ion channels. Furthermore, this sensitivity can be varied by the identity of subunits from which the pentameric receptor is formed. Thus there are subtypes of $GABA_A$ receptors that are insensitive to anaesthetics.[4]

Typical protein drug targets are as follows.

Carrier molecules

Ions and polar organic molecules require a carrier protein to transport them across the lipid cell membrane. Examples of therapeutic importance are the 5-hydroxytryptamine (5HT) and noradrenaline transporters, which are inhibited by the tricyclic and related antidepressant drugs,[5] and the proton pump, which is inhibited by omeprazole.[6] Omeprazole has been used for the prophylaxis of stress ulcer in intensive care units (ICUs), although a lack of detailed clinical trials has relegated it to a second-line drug.[7,8] Other examples of drugs used in ICUs that inhibit carrier molecules are the loop diuretics that inhibit the $Na^+/K^+/2Cl^-$ co-transporter and the cardiac glycosides that inhibit the Na^+/K^+ pump. There is increasing evidence of functionally distinct transporter subtypes, particularly amongst the amino acid neurotransmitter transporters such as GABA and glutamate[5] and these will be future targets for drug action.

Enzymes

Enzymes are a crucial part of most biochemical reactions. They may be inhibited reversibly, such as by neostigmine acting on acetylcholinesterase, or irreversibly, such as the inhibition of cyclo-oxygenase by aspirin. It is now known that many enzymes exist as multiple isoforms and the search is on for drugs having selectivity for one or more of these variants. Cyclo-oxygenase has two isoforms COX-1 and COX-2. COX-2 is induced in activated inflammatory cells and produces the prostanoid mediators of inflammation. COX-1, on the other hand, is expressed in most tissues and exerts many of the protective effects of prostanoids. Thus side effects of non-steroidal anti-inflammatory drugs (NSAIDs) could be reduced with the development of drugs that can cause selective COX-2 inhibition.[9] Many of the drugs used to treat infections in ICUs are enzyme inhibitors. A selection of these is listed in Table 3.1. Enzymes may also convert prodrugs into an active form such as the conversion of azathioprine to mercaptopurine or enalopril to

Table 3.1 Some enzyme inhibitors used to treat infections.

Drug	Enzyme inhibitor	Reasons for selectivity
Sulphonamides	Folic acid synthetase	Enzyme only essential in bacteria
Trimethoprim	Dihydrofolic acid reductase	Bacterial enzyme more sensitive to inhibition than mammalian enzyme
Aciclovir	DNA polymerase	Converted to active form by viral thymidine kinase that has greater affinity for the drug than the host enzyme
Zidovudine	Reverse transcriptase	Mammalian enzymes relatively resistant
Penicillin and cephalosporins	Transpeptidation enzyme necessary for cell wall synthesis	Not present in mammalian cells
Azoles (ketoconazole)	Fungal P450 enzymes responsible for ergosterol formation	Sterols not necessary in mammalian cells

enaprilat.[10] Both active drugs are also enzyme inhibitors, these being the enzymes involved in DNA synthesis and angiotensin converting enzyme, respectively. Enzymic conversion may also produce toxic metabolites, for example trifluoroacetic acid from halothane and N-acetyl-p-benzoquinone imine from paracetamol. Drugs may also be a false substrate for an enzyme. α-Methyldopa is converted to α-methylnoradrenaline[11] in the postganglionic sympathetic nerves. α-Methylnoradrenaline has greater selectivity for $α_2$-adrenoceptors than the normal metabolite, noradrenaline, and thus decreases blood pressure rather than raising it.

Ion channels

Voltage gated ion channels are membrane-spanning proteins that change shape depending upon the membrane potential. The consequences of the shape change is to open or close an aqueous pore in the centre of the protein which allows access of ions through the membrane dependent upon the transmembrane concentration gradient. A number of drugs can modulate the activity of these channels, some opening channels and others closing or blocking them. Many biotoxins are selective in this respect; tetrodotoxin, from the Japanese puffer fish or *fugu*, blocks sodium channels whilst scorpion α-toxin opens them.[12]

The most familiar example of drug-induced channel blockade are the actions of local anaesthetics on sodium channels. However, the characteristics of the block may depend upon the degree of ionisation (that is, ionic charge) of the molecule. Highly charged local anaesthetics require the channel to be open in order to gain entrance and produce blockade. The channel is open more often when the neurone is firing rapidly and thus the blockade will occur more rapidly in such conditions. This is known as use-dependent blockade. Neutral local anaesthetics, such as benzocaine, do not exhibit a use-dependent block.[13] Subgroups of sodium channels are now emerging which have differing sensitivities to drug action[12] and will provide another target for drug research.

Calcium channel blockers such as verapamil and nifedipine are also familiar drugs. These drugs are selective for L-type calcium channels that are important in smooth muscle contraction. Blockade of T-type calcium channels may be important in the anticonvulsant action of several drugs such as ethosuximide and flunarizine.[14] Potassium channel pharmacology is also rapidly expanding and we now know that the vasodilators minoxidil and diazoxide open the ATP-sensitive potassium channel and that the antidiabetic drug glibenclamide closes it.[15] Non-selective, voltage-sensitive potassium channel blocking agents include tetraethylammonium and 4-aminopyridine, but their clinical use is limited by excitatory side effects.[16] However, selective drugs acting on the voltage-sensitive potassium channels will certainly be revealed as time goes by. Some blockers of voltage gated ion channels are shown in Table 3.2.

Table 3.2   Voltage-sensitive channels.

Channels	Blockers
Calcium	
L	Nifedipine, diltiazem, verapamil
N	ω-Conotoxin GV1A
P	ω-Agatoxin 1VA high affinity
Q	ω-Agatoxin 1VA low affinity
T	Flunarizine, ethosuximide
Potassium	
K_A	4-Aminopyridine, tetrahydoaminocrine
K_V	4-Aminopyridine, charybdotoxin
$K_{V(r)}$	Dofetilide
$K_{V(s)}$	LY 97241
K_{SR}	Cs^+
Sodium	
I, II, III	Tetrodotoxin, saxitoxin
μ^1	Tetrodotoxin, μ-conotoxin
H_1	High-concentration tetrodotoxin, saxitoxin
PN3	Resistant to tetrodotoxin

Receptors

Receptors are defined pharmacologically as proteins that regulate a particular physiological role in response to recognition of a particular molecular shape. A typical example would be acetylcholine activating the nicotinic receptor and causing the contraction of skeletal muscle. The rest of this chapter concentrates on receptors that are the target of the majority of drugs in use at the present time.

Agonists and antagonists

The terms agonist (a molecule that binds to a receptor causing activation and resultant cellular changes) and antagonist (a molecule that attenuates the action of an agonist) only truly applies to receptors. These definitions can be further expanded.

Full agonist

A full agonist can produce the largest response that the tissue is capable of giving. The term efficacy[17] has been used to describe the way that agonists can vary in the response that they produce even when occupying the same number of receptors. A high-efficacy agonist will produce a maximum response even when occupying a small proportion of the available receptors.

Partial agonist

A partial agonist is an agonist that cannot fully activate the receptors irrespective of the concentration available. In contrast to a full agonist, a partial agonist cannot exert a maximal response. Buprenorphine is a partial agonist at opioid μ-receptors. Partial agonists have lower efficacy and cannot produce a maximal response even when occupying all the receptors.

Inverse agonists

The simplest definition is that the compound binds to a receptor but produces the opposite effect to an agonist. The best-described inverse agonists are the β-carboline derivatives at the benzodiazepine receptor.[18] Agonists at this receptor enhance GABA transmission, inverse agonists reduce GABA transmission, and antagonists have no effect on GABA transmission. Flumazenil, a benzodiazepine antagonist, will reverse the effects of both agonists and inverse agonists. However, this classification of individual drugs into agonists, antagonists, and inverse agonists may vary with the physiological state of the recipient. Flumazenil can provoke panic attacks in patients with panic disorders, but not in control subjects.[19] This suggests that flumazenil has partial inverse agonist activity in this subgroup of patients. Inverse agonists have now been described in many other receptor systems.[20]

In addition, the term inverse agonist has been used to describe a ligand that preferentially stabilizes inactive conformations of G-protein-coupled receptors.[21]

Competitive antagonists

A competitive or surmountable antagonist binds reversibly to the same receptor as an agonist, but occupies the site without activating the effector mechanism. A competitive antagonist has zero efficacy. Its action may be reversed by increasing the concentration of the agonist. The pharmacological effects seen after the administration of a competitive antagonist depends on the ongoing activity of the receptor system affected. For example, the autonomic nervous system is continuously active, so adrenoceptor or cholinoceptor antagonists cause significant changes in function. By contrast, in a fit unstressed person, opioid systems, for example, are rarely active and so an antagonist such as naloxone, when given alone, will have no discernible effect. This is not necessarily true in unhealthy individuals. Patients experiencing thalamic pain have been successfully treated with naloxone.[22]

Insurmountable antagonists

Once established, no amount of agonist will completely reverse the inhibition induced. If the antagonist binds covalently to the receptor, it may be possible to reverse it with competing agonists provided they are administered before the covalent bond has formed. Phenoxybenzamine is an insurmountable antagonist and covalently binds to α-adrenoceptors. Antagonists that bind to different sites on the receptor, causing a change in the conformation of the agonist-binding site (allosteric antagonism), are also insurmountable.

Receptor classification

Up until relatively recently, receptors were classified on the basis of drug-agonist effects and compounds that antagonised those effects. Classical experiments by Dale in 1913 showed that adrenaline caused vasoconstriction in some vascular beds and vasodilation in others. The former effect was blocked by an ergot derivative but not the latter. This observation was built on by others and allowed for a classification of α- and β-adrenoceptors.[23] Further agonist and antagonist discoveries allowed even greater subdivisions into α_1, α_2 and β_1, β_2 and β_3. The developing science of molecular biology demonstrated that receptors could also be classified according to their amino acid sequences and this has led to a profusion of receptors (α_{2A}, etc.),[24] although we still have no functional correlate for many of these. An annual update of known receptor classes is published in *Trends in Pharmacological Sciences, Receptor Supplement*.

Families of receptors

Four main families of receptors have been revealed by cloning and structural studies (see Figures 3.1 and 3.2).

Ligand gated ion channels

Several neurotransmitters convey their signals by directly opening ion channels and changing the cell membrane potential or ionic composition. These are usually involved in fast synaptic transmission and include the nicotinic cholinoceptor, $GABA_A$ and $GABA_C$ receptor for γ-aminobutyric acid, $5HT_3$ receptor for 5-hydroxytryptamine and the NMDA receptor for glutamate. They are multisubunit receptors in which all subunits traverse the membrane. Those most studied appear to be made up of five subunits,

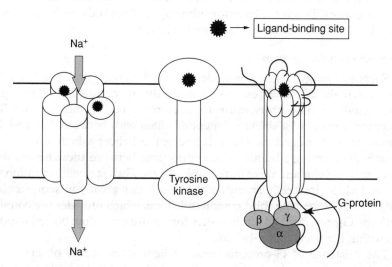

Figure 3.1 Membrane-bound receptors.

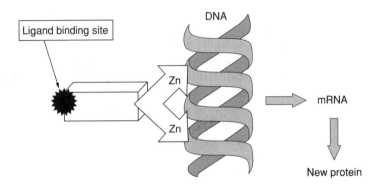

Figure 3.2 Intracellular receptor affecting gene transcription.

which may or may not be of the same type, surrounding a channel. The nicotinic receptor has four different subtypes (α, β, γ, δ) with two of the α type which bind acetylcholine being incorporated into the five-unit receptor.[25] By contrast, the GABA$_C$ receptor has five identical subunits.[2]

As with the voltage gated ion channels mentioned earlier, modulation of channel gating by the binding of ligands to a variety of sites on the receptor complex can significantly affect function, the benzodiazepine enhancement of chloride ion transport via the GABA$_A$ receptor being an important example. Indeed, the GABA$_A$ receptor may have 11 or more modulatory sites, making its pharmacology one of the most complex so far described.[2] There may be several variants of each subunit which, if incorporated into the receptor, can alter affinity, for not only the neurotransmitter itself, but also its modulators. This is the basis for subdivision of benzodiazepine receptors, the functional correlates of which are unclear.[26]

G-protein-coupled receptors

Receptors linked to guanine nucleotide-binding regulatory proteins or G-proteins, make up the largest proportion of the membrane-bound receptors and include adrenoceptors, muscarinic receptors, and opioid receptors. The receptor consists of a single polypeptide chain with between 300 and 500 amino acids arranged as seven connected α-helices which traverse the membrane forming a bundle. The connections between these helices form three extracellular and three intracellular loops. The extracellular amino terminal and the intracellular carboxy terminal vary greatly in sequence and length as does the long third cytoplasmic loop, which provides the coupling with the G-proteins. The binding sites for agonists are often buried in pockets within the bundle of α-helices.

The existence of G-proteins came to light when it was observed that stimulation of second messenger systems such as adenylyl cyclase required not only the receptor agonist but also the presence of guanosine triphosphate (GTP).[27] The G-protein was eventually isolated and found to be a heterotrimer with subunits called α, β, and γ in order of decreasing molecular weight.[28] The sequence of events following the agonist binding to the receptor is shown in Figure 3.3.

In its resting state the G-protein complex is not associated with any particular receptor and is freely diffusible in the plane of the membrane and can interact with several different receptor and effectors. Specificity for a particular agonist receptor complex always producing the same end biochemical change in the cell is guaranteed by the variability of the structure of the G-protein α-subunit. Many variants of the subunits have been described[29] and the number is still growing. Two bacterial toxins, pertussis and cholera toxins, have been particularly useful in helping to distinguish which type of G-protein is involved in a particular situation. Cholera toxin causes persistent activation of the G-protein that stimulates adenylyl cyclase (Gs) thus causing the excessive secretion of fluid from the gastrointestinal epithelium that is characteristic of the disease of cholera.[30] Pertussis toxin has no effect upon Gs but prevents the actions of other G-proteins such as Gi that inhibits adenylyl cyclase activity. Several G-proteins are

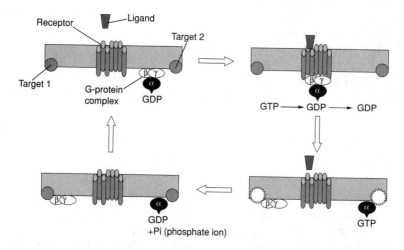

Figure 3.3 A diagrammatic view of the action of G-proteins. GDP, guanosine diphosphate; GTP, guanosine triphosphate. Targets 1 and 2 are two different G-protein effectors (see text). The agonist receptor complex causes a conformation change in the intracellular domain to a form which has high affinity for the G-protein. The process of binding the receptor to the G-protein catalyses the disassociation of guanosine diphosphate from the α-subunit of the G-protein and it is exchanged for intracellular GTP. This, in turn, causes the dissociation of the α-subunit from the β, γ-subunits. The latter two proteins appear to be involved in anchoring the protein to the plasma. They also have a signal tranduction function since some isoenzymes of adenylyl cyclase (see below) may be modulated by the combined β- and γ-subunits of the G-protein[31] and not by the α-subunit. The α-subunit modulates the action of a given effector, which, as we will see later, is not always adenylyl cyclase. The α-subunit has GTPase activity and converts GTP to GDP followed by reassociation with the other two subunits and the cessation of the signal.[32]

inhibited by pertussis toxin and thus its functional effects are less obviously explicable in terms of G-protein inhibition.

G-protein effectors (Figure 3.4)

Adenylyl cyclase is a membrane-bound enzyme that converts adenosine triphosphate (ATP) to cyclic 3,5-adenosine monophosphate (cAMP), which in turn activates protein kinase causing protein phosphorylation and a cellular response. One such response is increased activity of voltage-activated calcium channels in the heart, thus increasing the force of cardiac contraction (β-adrenoceptor activation via Gs protein). Adenylyl cyclase is inhibited by Gi-protein and this mechanism accounts for the inhibition of inflammatory pain by Gi-protein linked μ-opioid receptors.[33] Drugs can also affect the activity of adenylyl cyclase activity directly without the intervention of a receptor or G-proteins. Forskolin and fluoride ions are used experimentally to switch on adenylyl cyclase whilst methylxanthines, such as theophylline, inhibit the enzyme phosphodiesterase that normally breaks down cAMP.

Recent studies have described tissue-specific isoenzymes of adenylyl cyclase, each with unique patterns of regulatory response.[29] In addition, several types of phosphodiesterase have been described,[34] all of which could be future targets of drug action.

Phospholipase C is another membrane-associated enzyme which is activated by another subgroup of G-proteins identified as Gq.[35] This enzyme breaks down membrane phosphatidylinositol 4,5-biphosphonate into inositol 1,4,5-triphosphate [Ins $(1,4,5)P_3$] and diacylglycerol (DAG).

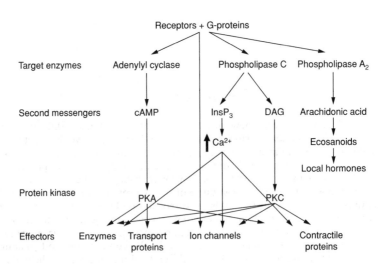

Figure 3.4 G-protein effectors. cAMP, cyclic 3,5-adenosine monophosphate; DAG, diacylglycerol; InsP$_3$, inositol triphosphate; PKA, protein kinase A; PKC, protein kinase C.

Ins(1,4,5)P_3 diffuses into the cell to release intracellular calcium that may initiate several processes such as secretion or contraction. Muscarinic receptors are known to be act via these pathways. Subsequently the Ins(1,4,5)P_3 is metabolised to give inositol, which can then be incorporated into membrane phospholipids to restart the cycle. Lithium, which is used to treat mania, has been shown to prevent the final metabolic step in the formation of inositol,[36] leading to the suggestion that mania is an overactivity of this system. DAG activates protein kinase C that is responsible for changes in ion channels, contractile proteins, enzymes, and transport proteins.[37] Isoenzymes of protein kinase C have now been identified, providing yet another target for drug action particular with respect to autoimmune diseases, transplant rejection, and oncology.[38]

Activation of phospholipase A_2 to release arachidonic acid also appears to be a G-protein-dependent process.[39]

Ion channels can be directly controlled by G-proteins by mechanisms that do not appear to involve adenylyl cyclase or any other second messenger system.[40] In the locus ceruleus, direct opening of potassium channels by G-proteins appear to occur when opioid receptors are stimulated.[41]

Direct enzyme-linked receptors

These receptors possess large intracellular and extracellular domains joined by a single membrane-spanning helix. The extracellular domain provides the binding site for peptide agonists, usually hormones that regulate differentiation, development, and growth. The intracellular domain is often a protein kinase that phosphorylates amino acid residues both of its own cytoplasmic domain and of target proteins.[42] Many phosphorylate tyrosine and the group has been called the tyrosine-kinase-linked receptors, of which receptors for insulin are a typical example. However, some receptors are serine/threonine kinase linked and others are linked to guanylyl cyclase, for example, the atrial natriuretic peptide.[43] The phosphorylated residues provide binding sites for other intracellular proteins (such as SH2 proteins) and eventually lead to altered gene transcription.[44] SH2 proteins contain the SH2 (or Src homology) domain which was first identified in the product of the *src* cellular oncogene. These proteins are now the target of much research, especially in the field of potential anticancer drugs.

Intracellular receptors affecting gene transcription

These non-membrane-bound receptors may either be nuclear (for example, thyroid hormone receptor) or predominantly cytosolic and form high molecular weight complexes with heat shock proteins (for example, glucocorticoid receptor).[45] In the latter, the presence of a ligand leads to the dissociation of the receptor from the complex and the movement of the receptor/ligand complex into the nucleus. It is obvious from the intracellular location of these receptors that ligands for these receptors must be lipid soluble and pass into the cell. The binding of the ligand to the receptor results in an uncurling of the receptor protein to reveal the DNA-binding domain. The DNA-binding domain consists of two "zinc fingers" which contain cysteine residues surrounding a zinc atom. These fingers are believed to wrap around the DNA helix at hormone-responsive elements in the strand. An increase in RNA polymerase activity and the production of a specific mRNA occurs and protein production is enhanced. A well-documented example of this is the increase in lipocortin production induced by glucocorticoid hormones. It has been suggested that lipocortin mediates the anti-inflammatory effects of glucocorticoids, but whether it is a primary mediator has been questioned.[46]

Factors changing responses to drugs

The responses of a patient to a drug may vary from patient to patient and may vary in a single patient with time.

Pharmacogenetics is the study of how variations in genetic makeup can affect drug action. Ethnic origins can be important in predicting drug responses;[47] Chinese, for example, differ from Caucasians in their high sensitivity to the cardiovascular effects of propranolol. Variations in plasma elimination half-time for various drugs such as coumarin anticoagulants and isoniazid are genetically determined. The presence of an atypical cholinesterase in patients exhibiting prolonged apnoea after suxamethonium has been particularly well studied.[48]

Over a period of time responses to a drug may be reduced as in tolerance or increased as in supersensitivity. These alterations in sensitivity may occur via several mechanisms.

- Pharmacokinetic changes such as altered absorption, elimination, or penetration to its site of action are discussed in detail elsewhere. These changes are particularly important when patients treated in ICUs where changes in liver and renal function are common.
- Compensatory homeostatic mechanisms can alter responses, particularly to hormone therapy, where there are negative feedback mechanisms. The diuretic effects of carbonic anhydrase inhibitors are transient because the acidosis caused reduces bicarbonate loss.
- Changes in receptors, especially those directly coupled to ion channels, can be rapid. This occurs at the neuromuscular junction where desensitisation is associated with a conformational change in the receptor such that it binds the agonist but the channel does not open in response.[49] Tolerance to agonists at β-adrenoceptors is associated with an inability of the agonist receptor combination to activate adenylyl cyclase. It has been suggested that phosphorylation of a single amino acid may be responsible for this change.[50] Tolerance to opioids has been linked to a failure of the receptor to couple to the G-protein, although this is probably only one of several mechanisms.[51]
- Changes in receptor number can also occur, but this process is usually slower than the uncoupling from second messenger described above. The

receptors for β-adrenoceptors and several peptides slowly reduce in number (down-regulation) in the presence of agonists. The receptors are believed to be taken into the cell by a process of endocytosis of patches of membrane. Down-regulation of β-adrenoceptors and $5HT_2$ receptors may be the basis of the action of antidepressant drugs.[52] These effects, like the development of antidepressant activity, take some weeks to occur. Up-regulation of D_2-dopamine receptors may be responsible for the emergence of tardive dyskinesia in patients on long-term neuroleptic drugs.[53]

- Mediators of drug action may become exhausted. A commonly quoted example is tachyphylaxis to indirectly acting sympathomimetics such as amphetamine. It produces its effects by releasing noradrenaline and other amines from nerve terminals and when these stores are depleted the drug becomes inactive. Abusers of the amphetamine derivative, Ecstasy, are being seen more frequently in ICUs[54] and these patients may have depleted biogenic amine reserves.

- Pathological disease states may also change pharmacodynamic responses to drugs as well as the pharmacokinetic handling mentioned above. Many are predictable from the known pharmacology of the drug. The cardiovascular depressant actions of the anaesthetic agents are greater in patients with diminished cardiac reserve. In addition, patients with obstructive airway disease may respond with exaggerated responses to ventilatory depressant drugs such as opioids. Such patients may also exhibit ventilatory depression in response to usually innocuous doses of benzodiazepines. Abnormally exaggerated responses to competitive neuromuscular blocking agents may be seen in patients with neurological diseases such as myasthenia gravis.

Most of this chapter has been devoted to the mechanisms of drug action in the normal individual with only brief attention to the disease state. It is worth emphasising that unexpected and unpredictable drug reactions and interactions are common in the critical care unit[55] and these will be dealt with in more detail in successive chapters.

1 Alton E. CF Gene therapy: where are we now? In Forum: UK Association of Pharmaceutical Scientists. *Pharm J* 1997;258:106.
2 Johnston GA. GABA_A receptor pharmacology. *Pharmacol Ther* 1996;69:173–8.
3 Parker RMC, Bentley KR, Barnes NM. Allosteric modulation of $5HT_3$ receptors: focus on alcohols and anaesthetic agents. *Trends Pharmacol Sci* 1996;17:95–9.
4 Franks NP, Lieb WR. Selectivity of general anaesthetics: a new dimension. *Nature Med* 1997;3:377–8.
5 Amara SG, Kuhar MJ. Neurotransmitter transporters: recent progress. *Annu Rev Neurosci* 1993;16:73–93.
6 Clissold SP, Campoli-Richard DM. Omeprazole: a preliminary review of its pharmacodynamic and pharmacokinetic properties and therapeutic potential in peptic ulcer disease and Zollinger–Ellison syndrome. *Drugs* 1986;32:15–47.
7 Lam NP, Le PD, Crawford SY, Patel S. National survey of stress ulcer prophylaxis. *Crit Care Med* 1999;27:98–103.
8 Tryba M, Cook D. Current guidelines on stress ulcer prophylaxis. *Drugs* 1997;54:581–96.

9 Mitchell JR, Akaarasereenont P, Thierermann C, Flower RJ, Vane JR. Selectivity of non-steroidal antiinflammatory drugs as inhibitors of constitutive and inducible cyclooxygenase. *Proc Natl Acad Sci USA* 1993;**90**:1 1693–7.

10 Rang HP, Dale MM, Ritter JM. How drugs act: molecular aspects. In: Rang HP, Dale MM, Ritter JM, eds. *Pharmacology*. Edinburgh: Churchill Livingstone, 1999:19–44.

11 Day MD, Rand MJ. Some observations on the pharmacology of α methyl dopa. *Br J Pharmacol* 1964;**22**:72–86.

12 Edwards G, Weston AH. Voltage-gated ion channels. In: Davis RW, Morris BJ, eds. *Molecular biology of the neuron*. Oxford: BIOS Scientific, 1997:145–73.

13 Wann KT. Neuronal sodium and potassium channels: structure and function. *Br J Anaesth* 1993;**71**:2–14.

14 Bean BP, Mintz IM. Pharmacology of different types of calcium channels in rat neurons. In: Peracchia S, ed. *Handbook of membrane channels: molecular and cellular physiology*. New York and London: Academic Press, 1994:199–210.

15 Edwards G, Weston AH. The pharmacology of ATP-sensitive potassium channels. *Ann Rev Pharmacol Toxicol* 1993;**33**:597–637.

16 Pomgs O. Structural basis of voltage gated K+ channel pharmacology. *Trends Pharmacol Sci* 1994;**13**:359–65.

17 Stephenson RP. A modification of receptor theory. *Br J Pharmacol* 1956;**11**:379–93.

18 Novas ML, Wolfman C, Medina JH, de Robertis E. Proconvulsant and "anxiogenic" effects of n-butyl β carboline-3-carboxylate, an endogenous benzodiazepine binding inhibitor from brain. *Pharmacol Biochem Behav* 1988;**30**:331–6.

19 Nutt DJ, Glue P, Lawson C, Wilson S. Flumazenil provocation of panic attacks. Evidence for altered benzodiazepine receptor sensitivity in panic disorders. *Arch Gen Psychiatry* 1990;**47**:917–25.

20 Milligan G, Bond RA, Lee M. Inverse agonism: pharmacological curiosity or potential therapeutic strategy. *Trends Pharmacol Sci* 1995;**16**:10–13.

21 Milligan G, Bond RA. Inverse agonism and the regulation of receptor number. *Trends Pharmacol Sci* 1997;**18**:468–74.

22 Budd K. Antagonists in anaesthetic practice. In: Atkinson RS, Adams AP, eds. *Recent advances in anaesthesia and analgesia*, vol 17. Edinburgh: Churchill Livingstone, 1992:157–72.

23 Alquist RP. A study of the adrenotropic receptors. *Am J Physiol* 1948;**153**:586–600.

24 Schwinn DA. Adrenoceptors as models for G protein-coupled receptors: structure, function and regulation. *Br J Anaesth* 1993;**71**:77–85.

25 Karlin A. Structure of nicotinic acetylcholine receptors. *Curr Opin Neurobiol* 1993;**3**:299–309.

26 Pleuvry BJ. Benzodiazepines: receptors and their ligands. *Curr Anaesth Crit Care* 1991;**2**:238–42.

27 Rodbell M, Birnbaumer L, Pohl SL *et al*. The glucagon-sensitive adenylyl cyclase system in plasma membranes of rat liver. V An obligatory role of guanyl nucleotides in glucagon action. *J Biol Chem* 1971;**246**:1877–82.

28 Gilman AG. G proteins and regulation of adenylyl cyclase. *J Am Med Assoc* 1989;**262**:1819–25.

29 Neer EJ. Heterotrimeric G proteins: organizers of transmembrane signals. *Cell* 1995;**80**:249–57.

30 Simon MI, Strathmann MP, Gautam N. Diversity of G-proteins in signal transduction. *Science* 1991;**252**:802–8.

31 Taussig R, Gilman AG. Mammalian membrane bound adenylyl cyclases. *J Biol Chem* 1995;**270**:1–4.

32 Gaziano MP, Gilman AG. Guanine nucleotide regulatory proteins: mediators of transmembrane signaling. *Trends Pharmacol Sci* 1987;**8**:478–81.

33 Levine JD, Taiwo YO. Involvement of the mu opioid receptor in peripheral analgesia. *Neuroscience* 1989;**32**:571–5.

34 Beavo JA, Conti M, Heaslip RJ. Multiple cyclic nucleotide phosphodiesterases. *Mol. Pharmacol.* 194; **46**:399–405.

35 Smrcka AV, Hepler GR, Brown KO, Sternweiss PC. Regulation of polyphosphoinositide-specific phospholipase C activity by purified Gq. *Science* 1991;**251**:804–7.

36 Berridge MJ. Inositol triphosphate, calcium, lithium and cell signalling. *J Am Med Assoc* 1989;**262**:1834–41.

37 Nishizuka Y. The family of protein kinase C for signal transduction. *J Am Med Assoc* 1989;**262**:1826–33.

38 Wilkinson SE, Hallam TJ. Protein kinase C: is its pivotal role in cellular activation over-stated. *Trends Pharmacol Sci* 1994;**15**:53–7.

39 Axelrod J, Burch RM, Jelsema CL. Receptor mediated activation of phospholipase A2 via GTP dependent proteins: arachidonic acid and its metabolites as second messengers. *Trends Neurosci* 1988;**11**:117–23.

40 Hille B. G-protein-coupled mechanisms and nervous signalling. *Neuron* 1992;**9**:187–95.

41 Koob GF, Bloom FE. Cellular and molecular mechanisms of drug dependence. *Science* 1988;**242**:715–23.

42 Fantl WJ, Johnson DE, Williams LT. Signalling by receptor tyrosine kinases *Annu Rev Biochem* 1993;**62**:453–81.

43 Ruskoaho H. Atrial natriuretic peptide: synthesis, release and metabolism. *Pharmacol Rev* 1992;**44**:479–602.

44 Mitchell RH. Second messenger pathways. In: Kendrew J, ed. *The encyclopedia of molecular biology*. Oxford: Blackwell Science Ltd, 1994 : 998–1002.

45 Chatterjee VKK. Steroid receptor superfamily. In: Kendrew J, ed. *The encyclopedia of molecular biology*. Oxford: Blackwell Science Ltd, 1994 : 1033–6.

46 Davidson FF, Dennis EA. Biological relevance of lipocortins and related proteins as inhibitors of phospholipase A2. *Biochem Pharmacol* 1989;**38**:3645–51.

47 Kalow W. Race and therapeutic drug response. *N Engl J Med* 1989;**320**:588–90.

48 McGuire MC, Nogueira CF, Bartes CF *et al.* Identification of the structural mutation responsible for the dibucaine resistant variant form of human serum cholinesterase. *Proc Natl Acad Sci USA* 1989;**86**:953–7.

49 Changeux JP, Giraudat J, Dennis M. The nicotinic acetylcholine receptor: molecular architecture of a ligand regulated ion channel. *Trends Pharmacol Sci* 1987;**8**:459–65.

50 Huganir RL, Greengard P. Regulation of neurotransmitter desensitization by protein phosphorylation. *Neuron* 1990;**5**:555–67.

51 Pleuvry BJ. Induction and prevention of tolerance to opioid drugs. *Curr Opin Anaesth* 1992;**5**:555–8.

52 Sulser F. Mode of action of antidepressant drugs. *J Clin Psychiatry* 1983;**44**:14–20.

53 Jenner P, Marsden CD. Adaptive changes in brain dopamine function as a result of neuroleptic treatment. *Adv Neurol* 1988;**49**:417–31.

54 MacConnachie AM. Ecstasy poisoning. *Intens Crit, Care Nurs* 1997;**13**:365–6.

55 Crispin PS, Park GR. Unexpected drug reactions and interaction in the critical care unit. *Curr Opin Crit Care* 1997;**3**:262–7.

4: Renal failure

JW SEAR

The administration of sedative, analgesic, and other drugs to the critically ill patient may result in untoward effect as a result of alterations in drug kinetics and dynamics. Often these effects occur through interactions between drugs or with the disease processes seen in the critically ill. This chapter considers the influence of renal impairment on drug handling and the dynamic effects of drugs in the critically ill.

Influence of renal disease on drug metabolism in the liver

There is little evidence in man that chronic uraemia results in impairment of hepatic drug biotransformation. However, uraemia can cause unusual drug responses (for example, due to intercurrent therapy – anaesthesia interactions; reduced plasma protein binding of drugs leading to increased free fraction and exaggerated responses; altered drug metabolite elimination; or reduced biotransformation due to low plasma pseudocholinesterase activity).

Chronic renal insufficiency may cause alterations in drug disposition through changes in plasma protein binding, altered cellular metabolism, and altered drug and metabolite elimination.

Basic drugs (that is, those with a pK_a >7·4; for example, etomidate, ketamine, diazepam and midazolam, morphine, pethidine, fentanyl, alfentanil and sufentanil) bind primarily to α_1-acid glycoproteins whereas acidic drugs bind to albumin. In uraemia, protein binding of basic drugs is unaltered, whilst there is a significant decrease in the binding of acidic compounds (for example, thiopentone, propofol).

The decrease in plasma protein binding is multifactorial and includes:

- low plasma albumin concentrations due to increased excretion (for example, in nephrosis), or decreased synthesis
- the influences of uraemia *per se* on the conformational structure of proteins due to the accompanying changes in blood pH, degree of ionisation, and hydrogen bonding. These factors may alter the structure and affinity of drug binding sites
- competition existing between drugs and their metabolites, and/or drugs and accumulated endogenous and exogenous substrates.[1]

50

In vitro studies suggest that chronic uraemia affects hepatic drug metabolism (oxidation, reduction and *N*-demethylation, and microsomal cytochrome P450 activity).[2,3] However, *in vivo*, uraemia has little effect on the major pathways of drug handling. Phase I oxidative metabolism is either normal or increased (possibly due to the increased free drug), whilst the activities of reductive and hydrolytic pathways are often reduced. Phase II conjugation reactions are unaltered (see later discussion related to the glucuronide conjugates of morphine). As a result of changes in protein binding and drug metabolism, the apparent volumes of drug distribution are increased, and there may be an apparent increase in total drug clearance. However, free drug clearance is usually unchanged in patients with renal failure. Preoperative use of haemodialysis or plasma ultrafiltration may lead to intravascular volume depletion and hence further alterations in drug disposition.

Effect of renal dysfunction on the handling and dynamic characteristics of drugs used in the critically ill

Sedatives and hypnotics

These drugs are widely used to decrease the level of consciousness and allay anxiety during the control of ventilation in the critically ill patient.

Barbiturates

Despite the increased sensitivity to barbiturates seen in patients with chronic renal impairment, thiopentone is still widely used for induction of anaesthesia. However, normal induction doses cause prolonged unconsciousness the duration of effect being related to the blood urea concentration.[4] Various suggestions have been made as to the cause of the increased sensitivity. These include increased blood–brain barrier permeability,[5] increased unbound barbiturate in uraemic patients,[6,7] qualitative plasma albumin abnormalities,[8] or abnormal cerebral uptake and metabolism of the barbiturate.[9]

The disposition of thiopentone in patients with renal failure has been studied by several authors.[6,7] The main findings are an unaltered total drug elimination half-life, but an increased free-drug fraction. No differences have been found, when compared to healthy patients, in the unbound drug volumes of distribution and systemic clearance (Table 4.1). The increased free-drug fraction will result in higher brain concentrations of thiopentone. However, there are no studies to date specifically examining the use of thiopentone by infusion for sedation in the critically ill patient with renal impairment. Pentobarbitone (an active metabolite of thiopentone) has different physicochemical and kinetic properties; it has advantages over the parent drug in that its kinetics are unaltered in renal failure.[10] There are no data on the disposition of methohexitone in patients with chronic renal failure.

51

Table 4.1 Influence of chronic renal failure on the disposition of intravenous induction agents (mean values, except where indicated)

	Patients with normal renal function				Patients with impaired renal function			
	$t_{1/2el}$	Cl_p	V_{ss}	FF	$t_{1/2el}$	Cl_p	V_{ss}	FF
Thiopentone								
1	611	3·2	1·9	15·7	583	4·5*	3·0*	28·0*
2	588	2·7	1·4	11.0	1069	3·9	3·2*	17·8*
Pentobarbitone								
3	1590	0·36	0·82	–	1278	0·57	0·99	–
Midazolam								
4	296	6·7	2·2	3·9	275	11·4*	3·8*	5·5*
Diazepam								
5	5540	0·3	2·1	1·4	2196*	0·9*	2·8	7·0*
Etomidate								
6	–	–	–	24·9	–	–	–	43·4*
Propofol								
7	1714	11·8	19·8	–	1638	12·9	22·6	–
8	–	–	–	0.98	–	–	a	1·11
							b	0·87
9	420+	33·5	5·8	–	513+	32·0	11·3*	–
10	1878	24·1	25·6	(mean values for ICU patients)				
11	1411	31·5	(range: 21·7–132·5 of clearance values in ICU patients)					

Source of data: 1, Burch and Stanski[6]; 2, Christensen et al.[7]; 3, Reidenberg et al.[10]; 4, Vinik et al.[11]; 5, Ochs et al.[12]; 6, Carlos et al.[13]; 7, Kirvela et al.[14]; 8, Costela et al.[15]; 9, Ickx et al.[16]; 10, Albanese et al.[17]; 11, Bailie et al.[18].
$t_{1/2el}$, elimination half-life (min); Cl_p, systemic clearance (ml/kg/min); V_{ss}, apparent volume of distribution at steady state (1/kg); FF, free or unbound fraction of drug (%); +, median values. * $p < 0.05$ vs healthy subjects. a and b, pre- and postdialysis.

Etomidate

There are no formal studies on the disposition or dynamics of carboxylated imidazole, etomidate, in patients with renal failure, although Carlos et al. have shown decreased plasma protein binding in patients with uraemia.[13]

Ketamine

Ketamine undergoes hepatic biotransformation with the formation of norketamine and dihydroketamine metabolites. The main route of drug elimination is via the kidney; hence administration of continuous infusions to the patient with renal impairment may lead to increased plasma concentrations of active metabolites (especially norketamine) and the glucuronide conjugates. Its use for sedation in the critically ill is limited because of its psychotomimetic side effects.

Propofol

This is the most widely used sedative in the critically ill patient who requires controlled ventilation in the intensive care unit (ICU). The disposition of bolus doses of propofol is unaltered in terms of terminal half-life and clearance in patients with renal failure, as is the degree of plasma protein binding.[14,15] Similarly prolonged infusions of propofol administered to patients undergoing renal transplantation are associated with disposition kinetics similar to those in healthy patients receiving the drug.[14] Unlike the barbiturates, no apparent differences in dose requirements exist between patients with normal or abnormal renal function.

Kirvela *et al.* have also shown similar cardiovascular changes following propofol 2 mg/kg preceded by fentanyl 3 μg/kg in adequately volume-loaded uraemic patients to those in healthy subjects.[14] There was significant vasodilatation in all patients, with falls in arterial blood pressure. Adequate antihypertensive therapy in the uraemic patients may have contributed to the cardiovascular stability. There are no apparent differences in dose requirements in critically ill patients with normal or abnormal renal function.[19,20]

In the critically ill, the disposition of propofol is unchanged, although prolonged infusions are associated with longer terminal-phase half-lives, and larger apparent volumes of distribution at steady state; clearance is unaltered.[17,18] The effect of haemodiafiltration on propofol sedation requirements in critically ill patients has been examined by Eddleston *et al.*[21] Although the introduction of filtration did not affect the dosing requirements of these patients, there was a reduction in blood propofol concentrations in seven out of nine patients, with arousal in three of the seven. Diafiltration had no further influence on dose requirements. The drug concentrations associated with adequate sedation ranged from 0·52 to 4·14 μg/ml. No significant prolongation of its sedative effect has been reported in patients with renal disease.

Benzodiazepines

Although these drugs have been widely used for sedation in the critically ill patient, current practice relates mainly to midazolam.

Midazolam Midazolam is widely used for sedation in the ICU, but its disposition may be altered in the critically ill patient.[22] It is a water-soluble benzodiazepine which normally has a short elimination half-life, as does its main metabolite, 1-hydroxymidazolam. If given by repeated increments or continuous infusion, recovery time may be prolonged in the presence of renal failure due to accumulation of active metabolites. More recently, the importance of the sedative properties of these metabolites of midazolam have been recognised. The first step in the metabolism of the imidazolino-benzodiazepine is by hydroxylation involving cytochrome P450 3A4 to 1-hydroxymidazolam and 4-hydroxymidazolam. These are then both conjugated to the corresponding glucuronides, and eliminated by glomerular filtration and tubular secretion. In end-stage renal failure, high concentrations of 1-hydroxymidazolam glucuronide accumulate, and in some patients may be responsible for prolonged sedation.[23,24] Bauer *et al.* have shown there to be *in vitro* binding of the glucuronide to the cerebral benzodiazepine receptor, suggesting it may have substantial pharmacological activity.[24]

Uraemia also increases the free-drug fraction (from 3·9% to 6·5%), and as a consequence there is a significantly greater total drug clearance and apparent volumes of distribution when compared with healthy controls. There are no differences in unbound drug kinetics, and the elimination half-life is similar in the two groups (4·6–4·9 hours).[11]

Because of the accumulation of pharmacologically active metabolites, Shelly *et al.* found that the time to awakening after sedation by midazolam infusion for periods between 1·8 and 9·5 days was 13·6 hours (range 0–58 hours) in patients with normal renal function compared with 44·6 hours (2–120 hours) in those with renal failure.[25] Such variability cannot be explained by alterations in the cytochrome P450 3A4 activity, and supports the data of the other authors mentioned above that the metabolites of midazolam are pharmacologically active.

Diazepam This sedative has an elimination half-life of about 30 hours, and is mainly biotransformed in the liver into the two active compounds desmethyldiazepam and oxazepam. The former metabolite has a longer elimination half-life (96 hours) than the parent drug; under steady state conditions, its plasma concentration may exceed that of diazepam itself. In patients with chronic renal failure, Kangas *et al.* demonstrated a decrease in the plasma protein binding of diazepam.[26]

In a more recent study of the disposition of diazepam in patients with chronic uraemia, Ochs *et al.* found both an increased volume of distribution and increased systemic clearance, both secondary to an increase in the free unbound drug fraction (from 1·4% to 7·9%).[12] There was no difference in free-drug clearance in the uraemic and healthy patients; although the former group had a smaller volume of distribution.

Other IV benzodiazepines Single-dose studies with lorazepam indicate no alterations in the terminal half-life in renal failure;[27] however, these same authors have described impaired drug elimination following chronic administration to two patients with uraemia.[28]

In summary, the most appropriate sedative options for the critically ill with renal impairment are either propofol by infusion or the benzodiazepine lorazepam (the latter being most conveniently administered by intermittent bolus dosing). The use of midazolam may be associated with prolonged recovery on cessation of the sedative. Although etomidate has the advantage of minimal cardiovascular and respiratory depressant properties, its long-term use has been associated with adrenocortical depression and increased mortality. There are no separate studies evaluating its use in the critically ill patient with renal impairment. The barbiturates (particularly thiopentone) are best reserved for the control of intracranial pressure or convulsions.

Opioids

In the healthy patient, most opioid drugs are metabolised to inactive compounds which are then excreted in the urine or bile, biotransformation accounting for between 80 and 95% of the elimination of pethidine, alfentanil, fentanyl, sufentanil, and morphine. Phenoperidine differs from these other opioids in that about 50% is normally eliminated in the urine in an unchanged form. Thus in renal failure, the action of phenoperidine is most likely to be prolonged.

Morphine

This is still the most widely used drug in the provision of pre- and post-operative analgesia, and we are still learning about its disposition in patients with renal failure.

Morphine is metabolised primarily by the liver, where it undergoes glucuronide conjugation to morphine-3-glucuronide (M3G, the main metabolite; 40%) and morphine-6-glucuronide (M6G, 10%). While the latter is a more potent analgesic than the parent drug,[29] M3G has been shown in animal models to antagonise both morphine and M6G.[30,31]

Mostert et al., Don et al., and Stanley et al. have all reported prolonged or exaggerated clinical effects when IV morphine was given to patients with chronic renal failure.[32-34] Olsen and his colleagues studied the plasma protein binding of morphine in healthy patients and those with renal failure. In uraemia, the free-drug fraction increased from 65% to 70-75%.[35] The development of high pressure liquid chromatography (HPLC) assays for morphine and its metabolites and of non-cross-reacting immunoassays has allowed the clinician to study the kinetics of single and multiple doses in patients with renal impairment.

The role of the kidney in the elimination of morphine is still unclear. There are, however, two lines of data that help us evaluate the problem further. In sheep, Sloan et al.[36] and Milne et al.[37, 38] have all reported that the kidney contributes to the total body clearance of the opioid in healthy animals. In a more recent paper, Milne et al. have examined the influence of renal failure on the disposition of morphine, M3G, and M6G following an intravenous infusion of morphine.[39] Renal failure was achieved in the sheep by removal of the right kidney and then infusion of polystyrene microspheres to the left kidney. Once renal failure was established, morphine was infused as a two-stage infusion for six hours. Total body clearance was unaltered when the data from these sheep were compared with data from the normal animals cited in Milne et al.[38]; however, the renal elimination of morphine was reduced from 0·83 to 0·25 l/min. The pulmonary arterial blood ratios of the AUC's (areas under the concentration–time curve) of M3G/morphine and M6G/morphine were 18·3 and 0·48 (compared with

6·8 and 0·18 in control animals). Thus in renal failure, similar morphine plasma concentrations were observed as in healthy controls for the same infusion regimen. However, M3G and M6G were increased. When the total body clearances of morphine were compared in those animals where there was pretreatment and renal failure data, there was a significant reduction in total body morphine clearance (from 2·1 to 1·5 l/min). There was also a significant association between the clearance of morphine by the kidney and its renal excretory clearance of creatinine ($r_s = 0·89$).

Our own data from patients with normal renal function and those in patients undergoing renal transplantation[40] concur with the findings of Aitkenhead et al.,[41] Sawe and Odar-Cederlof,[42] Woolner et al.,[43] and Chauvin et al.,[44] all of which demonstrate that renal failure has little effect on morphine clearance after IV bolus doses, but does result in the accumulation of both M3G and M6G. In patients undergoing renal transplantation and receiving 10 mg morphine IV as supplement to nitrous oxide–oxygen anaesthesia, we found that the elimination half-lives of M3G and M6G ranged between 300 and 920 minutes, and 220 and 900 minutes, respectively. These values compare with values between 100 and 320 minutes in our anaesthetised patients with normal renal function.

As in the sheep, chronic renal failure was associated with a larger AUC for morphine, M3G and M6G between 0 and 24 hours in our data[40] (Figure 4.1), and in the studies of Osborne et al.[45] These two papers,

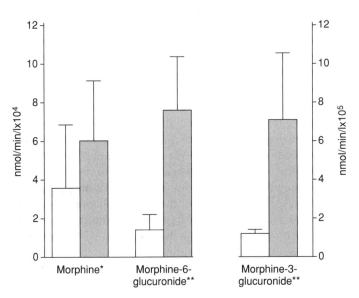

Figure 4.1 Areas under the concentration versus time curve for morphine, morphine-3-glucuronide, and morphine-6-glucuronide in anesthetised patients with normal renal function ($n = 5$) (open columns), and patients undergoing renal transplantation ($n = 11$) (shaded columns). (Adapted from [40]). *p<0.05; **p<0.01.

56

together with those of Mazoit et al.[46] and Sloan et al.[36] all offer support to the view that the kidney may itself have a role in morphine metabolism. Whereas the papers of Mazoit and Sloan suggest that around 30–35% morphine elimination may be by non-urinary excretion, non-hepatic degradation (that is, potentially by renal parenchymal metabolism), the two studies in patients with renal failure offer another explanation.

The increased plasma morphine concentrations (and larger AUC) could have occurred by hydrolysis of one or other of the accumulating glucuronides (probably the 3-glucuronide) back to the parent compound. This would tend to reduce the ratio AUC M3G: AUC M6G. There was a mean value in Osborne's study of around 5 in the healthy patients, and 3.9 and 4.5 in the groups of patients with end-stage renal disease.[45] The same ratios in our patients were 8 in the healthy anaesthetised patients and 9 in those undergoing transplantation,[40] that is, not different but again in keeping with the findings of Osborne, and probably due to the onset of renal drug elimination during the 24-hour study period.

More recently, Milne et al. have examined the relationship between renal creatinine clearance and the renal clearances of morphine, M3G, and M6G in 15 ICU patients with variable degrees of renal impairment.[47] For all three compounds, there was a linear relationship between free-drug clearance and creatinine clearance. The unbound clearance of morphine exceeded that of creatinine, whilst those of M3G and M6G were similar. The ratios of the plasma concentrations of M3G/morphine and M6G/morphine ranged between 4 and 170, and 0·79 and 51, respectively. Similar values have been reported by Petersen et al. in terminal cancer patients with impaired renal function receiving subcutaneous morphine.[48] The mean plasma concentration ratio of M3G: M6G was 5·0 (similar to the ratios of AUCs seen in the study by Osborne et al.[45] The unbound fractions for morphine, M3G, and M6G were 74%, 85% and 89% respectively the former figure being significantly greater than that determined by Olsen et al.[35]

In healthy volunteers, Loetsch et al. determined the half-lives of M3G and M6G to be of the order of 2·8–3·2 hours and 1·7–2·7 hours, respectively.[49] Thus, the longer half-lives of M3G and M6G (41–141 hours and 89–136 hours) reported by Osborne et al.[50] and Sawe and Odar-Cederlof[42] in patients with impaired renal function may be clinically important in the prolonged effect of the parent drug. Sawe has shown a significant correlation between the M3G half-life and the plasma urea concentration whilst we found a significant correlation between the half-lives of both M3G and M6G and the immediate postoperative 24-hour creatinine clearance in the patients undergoing transplantation ($r = 0·87$ and $r = 0·63$, respectively; $p<0·01$ and $p<0·05$). However, there are insufficient data at present to derive a nomogram relating plasma creatinine, predicted or measured creatinine clearance, and accumulation of the active M6G in the patient with renal impairment.

If an infusion of morphine is administered to patients with impaired renal function, accumulation of M6G may occur to give a clinical picture of a persistently narcotised patient.[50-52] The importance of the 6-glucuronide can also be seen in the case reported by Covington et al.,[53] where severe respiratory depression was observed in a patient with end-stage renal disease receiving morphine patient-controlled analgesia (PCA) for post-cholecystectomy pain. The blood morphine concentration was 73 ng/ml (within the therapeutic range), but the 6-glucuronide level was significantly elevated at 415 ng/ml. Similar data have been recently described by Carr et al.[54] where the PCA dose requirements after cadaveric renal transplantation ranged between 3 and 4·7 mg/h compared with 4·6–23·6 mg/h in patients with normal renal function undergoing lower abdominal surgery. The former group showed considerably greater AUCs for the active metabolite M6G.

In a further study examining morphine and metabolite transfer across the blood–brain barrier (BBB), 14 patients (8 healthy) were given a single dose of oral morphine (MST, 30 mg) before receiving continuous spinal anaesthesia for peripheral vascular or orthopaedic surgery.[55] Plasma concentrations of M3G and M6G were greater in the six patients with end-stage renal disease, as was the AUC (0–24 hours) for morphine. This latter observation could be explainable either by increased oral absorption, decreased elimination or increased enterohepatic circulation in renal disease. However, whereas CSF morphine concentrations were similar in the two patient groups, there was a greater BBB transfer of the two glucuronides in the renal failure patients. This is probably due to the higher plasma concentrations (and the greater than predicted lipophilicity of the glucuronides)[56] rather than an increased BBB transfer in the patient with renal failure. Unfortunately, this study did not address the key issue – whether the higher CSF concentrations of M6G were associated with greater respiratory depression, or sedation, or prolonged analgesia.

What is the contribution of M6G to the analgesic and depressant effects of morphine? In 14 patients with chronic pain (but normal renal function), Portenoy et al. assessed the contribution of the glucuronide to overall analgesia when produced by a morphine infusion.[57] Pain relief was greatest when the measured M6G/morphine molar ratio was > 0·7 : 1, with a significant correlation between the molar ratio and pain relief. There is a complex relationship between the drug's kinetic and dynamic profiles and the severity of the renal impairment. From a recent systematic review by Faura et al.,[58] one can see that there are wide ranges in the ratio of metabolites to morphine in the normal population (0·001–4 for M3G: morphine and 0–97 for M6G: morphine), depending on the dosing route. However, there is a high correlation in the plasma concentrations and plasma ratios for the two glucuronides despite a variety of clinical scenarios (for example, age, anaesthesia, renal disease), suggesting that there is only a single glucuronidating enzyme.

In the critically ill patient with renal failure, intermittent haemodialysis and filtration produce a considerable decrease in the plasma concentrations of morphine; a mean reduction of 75% (range 47–100%) following haemofiltration, and 48% (24–84%) following dialysis alone.[59] Both filtration and dialysis appear to extract morphine and M6G efficiently,[60] with a sieving coefficient in excess of 0·5. Whether there is equal elimination of morphine and M6G in these critically ill patients is open to further evaluation.

There are also data to suggest increased concentrations of another morphine metabolite (normorphine) may be responsible for myoclonic activity, but this has not been confirmed by other researchers.[61] Similar alterations in the disposition of codeine, dihydrocodeine, and propoxyphene (with active metabolite accumulation) have been observed in patients with renal failure.[62-64]

Whether the altered kinetics of morphine and its surrogates are the sole explanation of their prolonged dynamic effect is uncertain. Uraemia is itself associated with CNS depression and the increased sensitivity to CNS depressant drugs may also be due to increased receptor responsiveness, or increased meningeal and/or cerebral permeability.[65,66]

Fentanyl, alfentanil, and sufentanil

Because of the significant dynamic effects of morphine and its active metabolite M6G, some ICUs prefer to provide analgesia in the critically ill patient with renal impairment by drugs of the phenylpiperidine group.

The kinetics of the archetypal drug, fentanyl, have been studied in awake patients with end–stage renal failure undergoing haemodialysis.[67] Corall et al. found an increased apparent volume of distribution, and an increased systemic clearance.[67] There are fewer data in the anaesthetised or critically ill patient with renal impairment. Our own data[68] and those of Koren et al.,[69], Duthie,[70] and Koehntop and Rodman,[71] show no significant differences in the disposition of fentanyl in patients with renal failure undergoing transplantation when compared with age-matched healthy subjects undergoing lower abdominal surgery, although Koehntop et al. found an inverse relationship between the degree of azotaemia and fentanyl clearance. In two of the eight patients in his study, administration of fentanyl 25 μg/kg was followed by the need for postoperative ventilation for prolonged ventilatory depression. Uraemia also caused no alteration in fentanyl binding.[72]

In critically ill patients, the kinetics of fentanyl show wider inter-individual variability than in the normal population; Alazia and Levron[73] have reported elimination half-lives of 10–56 hours, and systemic clearances of 7·3–20·1 ml/kg/min. The plasma protein binding varied between 77·7 and 82·4%, in agreement with the data of Bower.[72]

With alfentanil, there is an increased free-drug fraction in patients with uraemia,[74,75] together with greater total drug clearance rates and volumes of distribution, but no differences in the free-drug volume of distribution or clearance. The metabolites of alfentanil are probably inactive, and hence this opioid has been successfully used as the analgesic of choice when given by repeat dosing or continuous administration to patients with renal impairment. Because alfentanil equilibrates rapidly across the blood–brain barrier, its narcotic effects peak within 1–2 minutes of a bolus dose; and it is easy to titrate when given by continuous infusion. Our recent understanding of some of the factors causing inter-individual variability in alfentanil clearance arises from different concentrations of microsomal CYP 3A3/4.[76] However in the post-transplant patient, Koehntop et al. have provided data that leads to confusion of the overall picture, as they have found increased alfentanil clearance in the presence of enzyme inducers (as might be expected) but not decreased by potential competitive inhibitors (such as erythromycin, midazolam, and some antifungals).[77] When given by infusion to critically ill patients, Sinclair et al. showed the considerable kinetic and dynamic variability in drug requirements (0·56–8·43 mg/h and plasma concentrations associated with adequate sedation and analgesia of 40–1063 ng/ml) (Figure 4.2).[78] We were unable to relate plasma concentration or dose requirements to the degree of renal impairment of the patients.

Similarly, uraemia has no effect on either the plasma protein binding or disposition of sufentanil.[79–81] There are, however, case reports of prolonged narcosis following preoperative administration of sufentanil to patients with chronic renal failure,[79,82] which are probably due to alterations in the dynamics of the opioid in the uraemic patient. However, unpublished data suggest that the concentration–effect relationship for sufentanil in anaesthetised patients with renal impairment differs from that in healthy subjects. We have found the Cp_{50} (plasma drug concentration associated with no response to noxious stimulation in 50% of patients) to be 0·29 ng/ml when sufentanil by bolus injection was used to supplement 67% nitrous oxide in healthy patients undergoing lower abdominal surgery, as compared with 0·13 ng/ml in patients with renal failure undergoing transplantation.

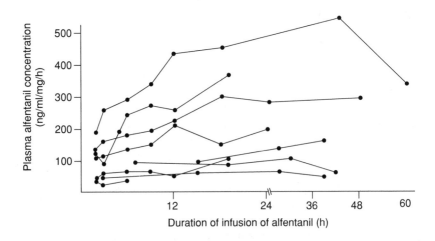

Figure 4.2   Plasma alfentanil concentrations (ng/ml) corrected to a uniform infusion rate of 1 mg/h in nine patients. (Adapted from[78], with permission).

The kinetics of the phenylpiperidine drugs and other opioids administered during anaesthesia to healthy and uraemic patients, or used in the critically ill, are shown in Table 4.2.

Table 4.2 Influence of chronic renal failure on the disposition of opioids in the anaesthetised patient (mean values except where indicated).

	Patients with normal renal function				Patients with impaired renal function			
	$t_{1/2el}$	Cl_p	V_{ss}	FF	$t_{1/2el}$	Cl_p	V_{ss}	FF
Morphine								
1	186	21·3	3·7	–	185	17·1	2·8*	–
2	307	11·4	3·8	–	302	9·6	2·4*	–
3	102	27·3	3·2	–	120	25·1	2·8*–	
4	210	11·5	2·8	–	191	10·3	1·8*	–
Fentanyl								
5	405	14·8	7·7	–	594*	11·8	9·5	–
6	–	–	–	20.8	–	–	–	22·4
7	–	–	–	–	382	7·5	3·1	–
8	1500	12·0	25·1	19.1 (mean values for ICU patients)				
Alfentanil								
9	90	3·1	0·3	11.0	107	3·1	0·4*	19·0*
10	120	3·2	0·4	10.3	142	5·3*	0·6	12·4*
Sufentanil								
11	76	12·8	1·3	–	90	16·4	1·7	–
12	195	18·2	3·6	7.8	188	19·2	3·8	8·6
Remifentanil								
13	4·0	33·2	0·19	–	4.9	35·4	0·25	–
Oxycodone								
14	138+	16·7+	2·39+	–	234+	12·7+	3·99+	–

Source of data: 1, Chauvin et al.[44]; 2, Sear et al.[40]; 3, Osborne et al.[45]; 4, Aitkenhead et al.[41]; 5, Duthie[70]; 6, Bower[72]; 7, Koehntop and Rodman[71]; 8, Alazia and Levron[73]; 9, Chauvin et al.[74]; 10, Bower and Sear[75]; 11, Davis et al.[80]; 12, Sear[81]; 13, Hoke et al.[83]; 14, Kirvela et al.[84].
$t_{1/2el}$, elimination half-life (min); Cl_p, systemic clearance (ml/kg/min); V_{ss}, apparent volume of distribution at steady state (l/kg); FF, free or unbound fraction of drug (%).
* $p < 0.05$ vs healthy subjects; + median values.

Remifentanil

Although remifentanil is a fentanyl derivative, its elimination depends not on the liver, but on hydrolysis of the methyl ester linkage by blood and tissue non-specific esterases. The clearance of remifentanil is high (25–45 ml/kg/min) and only minimally dependent on hepatic and renal function. The major metabolite is a primary carboxylic acid (GI 90921) which has a potency of about 1/4600 of the parent drug.

Recent studies with remifentanil have shown its kinetics to be substantially unaltered in patients with renal disease; there was no change in clearance or volume of distribution, although the elimination half-life was slightly prolonged.[83] However, the context-sensitive half-time is 3–4 minutes – even after prolonged infusions. Concentrations of the metabolite (GI 90921) showed a longer half-life (from 1·5 to >26 hours) and reduced clearance in the renal group when compared with healthy volunteers (the ratios of the AUC for GI 90921: remifentanil being 170–240 : 1 in the renal failure group compared with 6·3 : 1 in healthy subjects). At steady state, the concentrations of the metabolite were about 28–38 times higher than those in healthy people. At high infusion rates (>2 µg/kg/min), there is the possibility of some analgesic effect from the metabolite. Drug dynamics also appeared to be unaffected, with no increased respiratory sensitivity to the drug.[83]

Although there are reports of the use of remifentanil in the critically ill patient, there are insufficient safety data at present to allow comment on its use in the ICU patient with renal impairment.

Pethidine

There are few kinetic data on the disposition of pethidine in patients with renal impairment. In anaesthetised healthy patients, Mather *et al.* reported an elimination half-life of 186 minutes and clearance of 14 ml/kg/min.[84] Pethidine is mainly metabolised in the liver, with only 1–5% excreted unchanged in the urine. However, under acidic conditions (as may pertain in renal failure), the percentage of unchanged pethidine available for renal excretion may increase to 25%.[86] Recent data from Chan *et al.* support the view that systemic pethidine clearance is dependent on renal function.[87]

The dynamics of pethidine in chronic renal failure have recently been assessed by Burgess *et al.*[88] They have shown that patients with end-stage renal disease have a reduced ventilatory response to CO_2 compared with a healthy control group. The administration of pethidine (1 mg/kg subcutaneous) did not have any greater effect in the renal failure patients. Whether this observation is transferable from the laboratory to the ward scenario remains to be tested!

Just as with morphine, Szeto *et al.* have shown that when repeated doses of pethidine are given to patients in chronic renal failure, there is accumulation of the *N*-demethylated metabolite, norpethidine.[89] In one of these patients, the elimination half-life of norpethidine was 34·4 hours. The renal excretion of norpethidine is significantly correlated to the creatinine clearance rate,[90] as well as being pH dependent.[91] Under normal conditions, about 5–6% of a pethidine dose is eliminated as the nor-metabolite; but under acidic conditions, the amount may approach 30%. This metabolite has less analgesic, but greater convulsant activity than the parent drug,[92] and Szeto *et al.* have reported two patients in renal failure where increased plasma ratios of norpethidine/pethidine were associated with excitatory signs.[89] On these grounds, pethidine is probably best avoided as an analgesic drug in the critically ill patient with renal impairment.

There are few data on the effects of haemodialysis on opioid disposition. Turner et al. examined the extraction of morphine and pethidine, and found median values of 15% and 8% respectively,[93] suggesting that this route of drug elimination is unlikely to be clinically significant.

Phenoperidine is similarly contraindicated in the patient with renal failure, as it is metabolised to pethidine and hence also to norpethidine.

Other opioids

The disposition of buprenorphine in patients undergoing renal transplantation is similar to that seen in patients with normal renal function.[94] During renal transplantation, no metabolites were detected in the recipient's plasma. However, when buprenorphine was infused to provide analgesia and control of ventilation in critically ill patients, there were measureable plasma levels of norbuprenorphine and the 3-glucuronide. In the presence of renal failure, the former were increased by a median of four times, and the latter by a median of 15 times. The normetabolite has been shown to be a weak analgesic when assessed using the rat tail-flick test.

The kinetics of oxycodone have also been evaluated in uraemic patients undergoing renal transplantation.[84] Like morphine, this semi-synthetic opioid has probable active metabolites (viz. noroxycodone and oxymorphone). The kinetic profile showed a prolonged elimination half-life in the patients with end-stage renal disease – secondary to a significantly increased volume of distribution and reduced clearance. Although the plasma concentrations of noroxycodone were higher in the uraemic patients, and the excretion of oxycodone and its metabolites was impaired, there was no reduced excretion of conjugated oxycodone and noroxycodone. Thus the use of oxycodone as an analgesic in patients with impaired renal function would also appear to be contraindicated due to active metabolite accumulation.

The handling and dynamics of both codeine and dihydrocodeine have been examined in patients with renal impairment; Guay et al. showed that the elimination half-life of codeine was increased from 4 to 18·7 hours in patients on haemodialysis.[64] In the presence of renal dysfunction, both Levine and Matzke et al. have described cases where conventional doses of codeine have resulted in narcosis.[95,96] The extent of the renal clearance of dihydrocodeine by the body is not known, but again prolonged narcosis in patients with renal impairment has been described by Barnes et al. and Redfern.[63,97] Barnes et al. found a similar elimination half-life for dihydrocodeine in normal and renally impaired patients, but greater peak plasma concentrations and AUC after oral dosing in the renal group. This suggests that in renal failure there is either a reduced systemic clearance or an increased oral bioavailability.[63]

In practice, most patients in the ICU in the UK receive either morphine, fentanyl, or alfentanil by infusion as analgesia. The use of remifentanil has been described in some specific patient groups (for example, following coronary artery bypass surgery).[98,99] Because of its short duration of action and rapid clearance, coupled with the short blood–brain equilibration half-time (1·5–3 minutes), remifentanil is best administered by titration to effect. Both codeine and dihydrocodeine, as well as morphine, oxycodone, and pethidine, are metabolised to active compounds; and should therefore best be avoided.

Despite its active metabolites, the Task Force of the American College of Critical Care Medicine and Society of Critical Care Medicine have recommended morphine as the preferred analgesic with titration of dose to effect.[100] In patients with haemodynamic instability or symptoms of histamine release, fentanyl (or alfentanil or sufentanil) may be used. An alternative is hydromorphone which has greater sedative but less euphoric properties than morphine. Pethidine (meperidine) is not recommended because of the excitatory properties of the metabolite norpethidine. The use of partial agonist drugs is not supported by large clinical trials.

Neuromuscular relaxants

In general, the neuromuscular relaxants are a group of ionised, water-soluble compounds that are freely filtered at the glomerulus. The degree of protein binding of most relaxants is low (<50%) and hence changes in plasma protein concentrations (and hence binding) are unlikely to affect these drugs' kinetics to any great extent. However, if the drug is normally excreted unchanged through the kidney, then their kinetics (and more importantly their dynamics) will be altered in the critically ill patient with renal dysfunction. Table 4.3 lists the extent of urinary excretion in the elimination of the various muscle relaxants.

Table 4.3   Renal excretion of neuromuscular blocking drugs (expressed as a mean percentage (or range) of total drug elimination).

Drug	Excretion
Quaternary amines	
Suxamethonium	<10
Gallamine	>95%
Benzylisoquinolinium compounds	
d-Tubocurarine	31–45%
d-Methyltubocurarine	42–52%
Atracurium	10%
Doxacurium	25–30%
Mivacurium	<10%
Cis-atracurium	?
Aminosteroid compounds	
Pancuronium	35–50%
Vecuronium	15–20%
Pipecuronium	38%
Rocuronium	9%
Rapacuronium	30%

Depolarising neuromuscular relaxants

Although Wyant reported a decrease in the activity of the enzyme pseudo-cholinesterase (and hence a decreased rate of degradation of suxamethonium) in patients being treated for renal failure by haemodialysis,[101] this does not appear to be a significant problem with current haemodialysis techniques. Prolongation of the action of suxamethonium is seen in some patients with chronic renal failure, but the exact incidence is unknown. The second and more important problem is suxamethonium-induced increases in serum potassium concentrations. Way *et al.* showed the increase in potassium in patients on haemodialysis to be comparable with that seen in normal healthy individuals.[102] Pretreatment with non-depolarising neuro-muscular blocking drugs do not prevent this increase in plasma potassium concentrations.

For rapid sequence intubation in the critically ill patient, suxamethonium still remains the drug of choice, although large doses of non-depolarising agents (such as atracurium, *cis*-atracurium, rocuronium, rapacuronium and mivacurium) may offer an alternative in the significantly hyperkalaemic patient.

Non-depolarising or competitive neuromuscular relaxants

In the critically ill patient, prolongation of clinical effect due to altered kinetics (or accumulation of metabolites) is less relevant than when it occurs at the end of surgery. However, consideration of drug kinetics can lead to this problem being prevented.

The following drugs show significant alterations in duration of effect in renal failure.

d-Tubocurarine In healthy patients, about 70% of an IV dose is recoverable from the urine. However, if renal failure occurs, there is a compensatory increase in the extent of biliary excretion. Thus, in anaesthetised patients with chronic renal failure, prolonged paralysis is normally seen only after administration of large or frequent doses of the relaxant.[103] The duration of response to the drug is primarily determined by redistribution, with a terminal half-life in healthy patients of approximately 80 minutes (Table 4.4). Studies by Matteo *et al.* and Miller *et al.* have shown a decreased plasma clearance, and hence a slower decline in the plasma drug concentration in patients with renal failure.[104,105] Several cases of prolonged paralysis have been reported with use of *d*-tubocurarine in patients with renal failure undergoing surgery, but there are few data on use of the drug to provide relaxation in the critically ill subject requiring long-term paralysis for ventilation.

d-Methyltubocurarine A significant decrease in the systemic clearance of *d*-methyltubocurarine in patients with chronic renal failure has been reported by Brotherton and Matteo[106] and therefore this agent is best avoided in patients with renal failure.

Table 4.4 Disposition of neuromuscular blocking drugs in patients with chronic renal failure (mean values except where indicated).

	Patients with normal renal function			Patients with impaired renal function		
	$t_{1/2el}$	Cl_p	V_{ss}	$t_{1/2el}$	Cl_p	V_{ss}
1 DTC	152	–	–	256	–	–
2 DMTC	315	1·2	0·47	640*	0·4*	0·35
3 GALI	131	1·2	0·23	752*	0·2*	0·29
4 PANC	104	1·1	0·15	489*	0·3*	0·24
5	133	1·8	0·34	257	0·6*	0·33
6 ATRAC	21	6·1	0·19	24	6·7	0·26
7	17	5·9	0·14	21	6·9	0·21
8 CisATRAC	30	4·2	–	34	3·8	–
9 VEC	53	5·3	0·2	83*	3·2*	0·24
10 MIVAC:						
cis–cis	68	3·8	0·23	80	2·4*	0·24
cis–trans	2·0	106	0·28	4·3	80	0·48
trans–trans	2·3	57	0·21	4·2	47	0·27
11 RAPACUR	175	9·4	0·41	174	6·4	0·34
12 PIPERC	137	2·4	0·31	263*	1·6*	0·44
13 DOXAC	99	2·7	0·22	221*	1·2*	0·27
14 ROCUR	71	2·9	0·26	97	2·8	0·21

Sources of data: 1, Miller et al.[105]; 2, Brotherton and Matteo[106]; 3, Ramzan et al.[107]; 4, McLeod et al.[108]; 5, Somogyi et al.[109]; 6, Fahey et al.[110]; 7, de Bros et al.[111]; 8, Eastwood et al.[112]; 9, Lynam et al.[113]; 10, Head-Rapson et al.[114]; 11, Szenohradszky et al.[115]; 12, Caldwell et al.[116]; 13, Cook et al.[117]; 14, Szenohradszky et al.[118].
Kinetic parameters as in Tables 4.1 and 4.2; *$p < 0.05$.
DMTC, d-methyltubocurarine; GALL, gallamine; PANC, pancuronium; ATRAC, atracurium; CisATRAC, cis-atracurium; VEC, vecuronium; MIVAC, mivacurium; RAPACUR, rapacuronium; PIPERC, pipecuronium; DOXAC, doxacurium; ROCUR, rocuronium.

Gallamine Mushin et al. and Feldman et al. showed that between 85 and 100% of this drug was excreted by the kidney in man[119,120] and there are case reports of inadequate reversal or prolonged paralysis after its use in patients with renal insufficiency. In a recent kinetic study, Ramzan et al. found considerable prolongation of the elimination half-life of gallamine in patients with renal failure.[107]

Pancuronium In healthy patients, about 40% of an IV dose is excreted in the urine, and another 10% in the bile. Augmentation of biliary excretion occurs in renal failure, but there is still a decrease in systemic clearance of pancuronium[108,109,121] coupled with prolonged neuromuscular blockade.[122]

The following drugs show little effect of renal failure on their kinetics or dynamics.

Atracurium Initial clinical studies by Hunter *et al.* showed no difference in the duration of neuromuscular blockade from an initial dose of atracurium or from repeated doses when the drug was administered to patients with normal function and compared to patients who were anephric.[123] This was confirmed in dynamic–kinetic studies by Fahey *et al.* and de Bros *et al.* who demonstrated that onset time, duration of action, recovery time (from 25% to 75% initial twitch height), and disposition kinetics were unaltered in patients with renal failure.[110,111] A second study from Hunter *et al.* compared the properties of atracurium, vecuronium, and *d*-tubocurarine in healthy patients and those with renal failure.[124] Atracurium and vecuronium were little affected by renal failure but *d*-tubocurarine was longer acting and less predictable.

Atracurium has been administered by continuous infusion to maintain neuromuscular blockade in patients with renal failure, with rapid recovery reported following its use in this way and no differences between healthy and renal failure patients.[125,126] However, Nguyen *et al.* have observed a prolonged recovery rate and longer time to 90% recovery of twitch height when administering atracurium by infusion to anephric patients.[127]

Atracurium undergoes elimination by both Hofmann degradation and ester hydrolysis, although Fisher *et al.* have recently suggested that up to 50% of total systemic clearance cannot be accounted for by either of these mechanisms.[128] An important metabolite of atracurium, laudanosine, has been reported in animals to cause excitatory EEG activity when administered in high doses.

One of the major problems with atracurium in the critically ill patient could therefore be the accumulation of one or more of these metabolites. Yate *et al.*, Ward *et al.*, and Parker *et al.* all investigated the relationship between renal function and plasma concentrations of laudanosine.[129–131] With single doses of atracurium (0·3 mg/kg) there were no effects of renal failure on the disposition of atracurium or its two metabolites, laudanosine and the associated monoquaternary alcohol.[130] Peak laudanosine concentrations were not significantly different in healthy patients and those with renal failure, and in both groups, plasma laudanosine concentrations were considerably lower than those associated with EEG excitation in the anaesthetised dog (of the order of 17 µg/ml).[132] In ICU patients receiving atracurium by infusion, both Yate *et al.* and Parker *et al.* measured plasma laudanosine concentrations and found that it did not exceed 5·1 µg/ml[129,131] In the latter study, a constant rate infusion of atracurium (0·6 mg/kg/h) was used to aid ventilation in addition to sedative and analgesic drugs. The accompanying plasma laudanosine concentration plateaued at about 1·5 µg/ml in patients with normal renal function; but in those patients with acute renal failure, there was greater variability in laudanosine concentrations, with maximal values of 4·3 µg/ml (Figure 4.3).

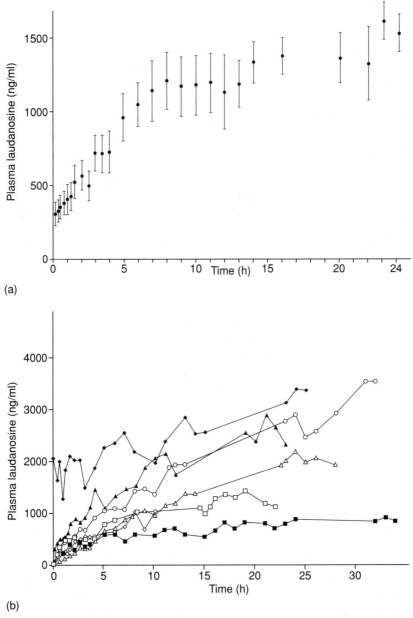

(a)

(b)

Figure 4.3 Plasma concentrations of laudanosine (ng/ml) for (a) seven patients with normal renal function (shown as mean ± sd) and (b) seven renal failure patients (shown as individual plots). (Reproduced with permission of authors and publishers.)[131]

The elimination of laudanosine is normally via the kidney, and in healthy subjects its half-life was increased from about 180 minutes to 374 minutes when given by infusion rather than as a bolus dose.[133] In acute renal failure, the elimination half-life was even greater, with a mean value of 1418 minutes. This may indicate that although the kidney is clearly important in laudanosine elimination, other organs (such as the liver) may also be involved.

In a separate study by Shearer et al. in critically ill patients requiring artificial ventilation (but with normal renal function), the urinary clearance of atracurium was 0·55 ml/kg/min, and that of laudanosine 0·33 ml/kg/min.[134] In seven other critically ill patients with renal failure, clearances of the two compounds in the haemofiltrate fluid were 0·11 and 0·09 ml/kg/min, respectively. Plasma clearances were not significantly different from those in the patients with normal renal function. Thus, normally about 9% of the laudanosine is excreted in the urine, and a smaller fraction (2%) in the haemofiltration fluid. Neither the parent drug nor its main metabolite are effectively removed by haemodialysis; elimination half-lives for laudanosine of up to 34·5 hours have been described by Hunter in patients receiving the neuromuscular blocking drug whilst undergoing haemofiltration.[135]

Vecuronium Evaluation of the kinetics of 0·1 mg/kg vecuronium in patients receiving cadaveric renal allografts and a control group of healthy patients was undertaken by Lynam et al.[113] Anaesthesia was maintained with nitrous oxide in oxygen and 1% end-tidal isoflurane. In the patients with renal failure, the duration of neuromuscular blockade and recovery from blockade were significantly prolonged. However, there were no significant kinetic differences (clearance, elimination half-life).

A number of reports have suggested that there may be accumulation of vecuronium in the patient with renal failure.[136–139] Because of the clinical importance of any dynamic interaction with renal failure, Beauvoir et al. conducted a meta-analysis of the available data.[140] Based on six studies, they found a significant increase in the duration of effect (as assessed to the time from injection to 25% recovery of twitch height) but no differences in onset time or 25–75% recovery times. However, the authors offered no firm aetiology for this effect.

There are several reports of the use of vecuronium to provide neuromuscular blockade in the critically ill patient.[141,142] In an isolated case report of an elderly patient with renal failure and subclinical chronic hepatic cirrhosis, Lagasse et al. describe prolonged neuromuscular blockade for 13 days after a three-day infusion at 0·13 mg/kg/h. There was no effect of haemodialysis on the degree of blockade.[143]

The metabolism of vecuronium by hepatic hydrolysis yields three desacetyl metabolites: 3-, 17-, and 3,17-desacetylvecuronium. The former of these is estimated to have the potency of about 80% of the parent drug, and there is good evidence that the 3-desacetyl metabolite accumulates in patients with renal failure.[142,144] Further recent studies by Segredo et al. propose that after prolonged dosing there may be distribution of drug into a large peripheral kinetic compartment with a low blood volume.[145] Caution should therefore be exercised to ensure complete return of neuromuscular function if multiple increments or prolonged infusions of the drug are used, especially in anephric patients.

Newer neuromuscular blocking drugs

There are six new neuromuscular blocking agents which show different disposition profiles in renal failure:

Pipecuronium This is a bisquaternary aminosteroid compound, which is mainly eliminated unchanged by the kidney. Renal failure causes a prolonged elimination half-life and reduced clearance.[116] There are no published data on its use in critically ill patients with renal dysfunction.

Mivacurium This is a short-acting benzylisoquinolinium compound which is metabolised by plasma esterases and presumably also in the liver. In healthy subjects, de Bros *et al.* demonstrated an elimination half-life of 17 minutes, and a clearance of 54 ml/kg/min;[146] the pharmacokinetics and duration of effect are not prolonged in renal failure.[147] Like atracurium, mivacurium has a number of stereoisomers (*cis–trans* 37%; *trans–trans* 57% and the less active *cis–cis* 6%). Head-Rapson *et al.* have examined the kinetics and dynamics of these three isomers in anaesthetised patients with renal failure.[114] Clearance of the *cis–cis* isomer was significantly reduced in renal failure; the disposition of the other two isomers was not altered. The clearance of each isomer correlated significantly with plasma cholinesterase activity. The median infusion rate required to achieve a common level of neuromuscular blockade (T_1/T_0 10%) was similar in patients with renal failure and in healthy subjects. However, Phillips and Hunter have demonstrated a prolonged duration of action in renal failure patients when compared with those with normal renal function,[148] probably due to lowered plasma cholinesterase activity.

Doxacurium This is a long-acting drug with an elimination half-life of 99 minutes, and clearance of 2·7 ml/kg/min. It is mainly excreted unchanged by the kidney, although esterase hydrolysis may contribute in part to the termination of drug effect. Clearance is reduced in patients with renal failure, with accompanying prolongation of effect.[117,149]

In a comparison with pancuronium in critically ill patients, Murray *et al.* found doxacurium to be well tolerated without evidence of tachycardia and with a relatively prompt recovery profile.[150] In contrast to pancuronium, doxacurium showed no inverse relationship after infusions of up to 2·6 days between recovery to the return of the fourth twitch of the train of four and creatinine clearance (Figure 4.4).

Rocuronium (ORG 9426) This is another agent with a rapid onset of effect and intermediate duration of action. Being a steroid molecule, it is metabolised in the liver, with only 9% of the injected dose being recoverable from the urine over the first 60 hours after administration. In a study com-

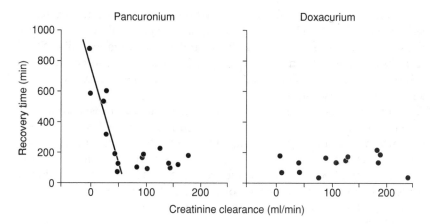

Figure 4.4 Recovery times versus two-hour creatinine clearance for patients receiving an infusion of pancuronium or doxacurium. The correlation of recovery time versus a creatinine clearance of <50 ml/min for patients receiving pancuronium is plotted. Some of the points represent more than one patient's values. (Reproduced with permission of the authors and publishers.[150])

paring its kinetics and dynamics in healthy anaesthetised subjects, and patients undergoing cadaveric renal transplantation, Szenohradszky et al. showed renal failure to alter drug distribution, but not systemic clearance.[118] In a separate study from Khuenl-Brady et al.[151] the dynamic characteristics of rocuronium were assessed during isoflurane anaesthesia in healthy patients and those with chronic renal failure. There were no differences in onset, duration of effect, or recovery after doses of 0·6 mg/kg and three maintenance doses of 0·15 mg/kg.[151] However, Cooper et al. have found both a decreased clearance of the relaxant in patients with renal failure during isoflurane anaesthesia, but no significant differences in drug dynamics.[152]

In a study of 32 ICU patients, Sparr et al. found no differences in rocuronium disposition after prolonged administration, nor differences in drug recovery times when compared with those seen after moderate duration infusions to surgical patients.[153] The exact implication of these findings must remain open to debate, as the patients studied had a wide range of creatinine clearances (27–186 ml/min). Further studies are clearly needed to define the properties of this neuromuscular blocking drug in the critically ill.

Thus, despite the chemical similarities of rocuronium to vecuronium, the former has a possible role in providing neuromuscular blockade to renally impaired patients.

Cis-atracurium This is one of the 10 stereoisomers of atracurium, and has the advantage of being three times more potent and releasing less histamine in animals. Unlike the parent compound, its metabolism is mainly by

71

Hofmann degradation with no ester hydrolysis. Recent studies by Kisor *et al.* confirm that the Hofmann pathway accounts for about 77% of total body clearance, organ clearance 23%, and renal clearance 16%.[154] The drug has an elimination half-life of 23 minutes, and clearance in healthy subjects of about 5·2 ml/kg/min. The main metabolites are laudanosine and a monoquaternary acrylate.

Two recent studies have examined the dynamics and disposition of *cis*-atracurium in renal failure. Boyd *et al.* found that at a dose of $2 \times ED_{95}$ (0·1 mg/kg), onset times were longer in the renal failure group, but recovery was not affected.[155] In these patients, the clearance of *cis*-atracurium was decreased by 13% and the half-life was longer (34·2 versus 30 minutes). Although plasma concentrations of laudanosine were elevated in patients with renal failure, the values were about one-tenth of those seen after atracurium.[112]

Rapacuronium (ORG 9487) This is another steroidal neuromuscular block-ing agent, but unlike some of the other newer compounds, it has a low potency. However, it has two advantages: very rapid onset of effect and a short duration of action. Hence it might be an appropriate drug to use in the critically ill where use of suxamethonium is contraindicated (for exam-ple, in the presence of hyperkalaemia). In doses of 1·5–2·5 mg/kg, complete blockade of the adductor pollicis muscle occurs in between 60 and 90 sec-onds with recovery to 25% of the first twitch of a "train-of-four" (TOF) at between 13 and 25 minutes. After prolonged administration, there is a decreased recovery rate, probably due to the accumulation of the active metabolite ORG 9488.[156]

In a recent study, Szenohradszky *et al.* have evaluated the kinetics and dynamics of rapacuronium in the patient with renal dysfunction.[115] They found small decreases in clearance and apparent volume of distribution in renal failure patients, but the dynamics of a single dose of 1·5 mg/kg were unaffected. However, clearance of the metabolite was decreased by 85%, indicating that there is likely to be a prolonged effect of the drug following repeated dosing in the patient with renal failure.

Infusions of neuromuscular blocking drugs in the critically ill patient

There are only a few studies that examine the effects of altered renal function in critically ill patients on the disposition of and dynamics of neuromuscular blocking drugs. In a small comparative study of 12 patients, *cis*-atracurium has been evaluated against atracurium. The population kinetic values for *cis*-atracurium and the three groups of atracurium isomers were in keeping with published data, but the *cis*-atracurium group of six patients showed smaller AUC and peak laudanosine concentrations.[157] After infusion times of 37·6 and 27·5 hours, respectively, at mean infusion rates of 0·19 mg/kg/h and 0·47 mg/kg/h, the recovery times to TOF >70% were similar in the two groups (at around 60 minutes).

A second key study is that of Prielipp *et al.*, who compared the infusion requirements and recovery profiles of vecuronium and *cis*-atracurium in the ICU.[158] In the 58 patients included, the mean infusion rates of the two neuromuscular blocking drugs were 0·9 μg/kg/min and 2·6 μg/kg/min, respectively. The durations of infusion were 66 and 80 hours, and recovery to TOF >70% was 387 and 68 minutes. Of more importance were the numbers of patients showing prolonged recovery (TOF <70% at 120 minutes after cessation of infusion): 15/58 patients, 13 having received vecuronium. Segredo *et al.* had previously also shown accumulation of vecuronium and its metabolites after infusion to the critically ill patient in the absence of renal impairment.[159] In a further study by the same group, a population kinetic study in six critically ill patients receiving vecuronium failed to show any significant effect of renal function on drug handling.[160] Other reports confirm the tendency for prolonged muscle weakness in the absence of high plasma drug concentrations (although clearly such values do not reflect the drug concentration at the affected site).[161,162] These papers all confirm the tendency for long-term use of neuromuscular blocking drugs (and particularly the aminosteroid relaxants) to be associated with post-infusion muscle weakness.

Thus, of these newer neuromuscular blocking drugs, *cis*-atracurium and rocuronium would appear suitable alternatives to atracurium in critically ill patients with renal impairment. Mivacurium and vecuronium are both probably best avoided in the critically ill ICU patient. Potentiation of neuromuscular blockade by any of the relaxants may occur in ill patients due to an associated metabolic acidosis. In the uraemic patient, potentiation of blockade may also occur due to hypokalaemia, hypocalcaemia, hypermagnesaemia, parenteral or topical use of some aminoglycoside antibiotics, frusemide, mannitol, and methylprednisolone.

Antibiotics

In the critically ill patient, appropriate antibiotic therapy may require administration of drugs with narrow therapeutic margins, and hence liability to toxic side effects. Examples of some of these side effects are shown in Table 4.5. The effects of aminoglycosides on the kidney can be potentiated by the associated administration of diuretics such as frusemide.

Many antibiotics are eliminated through the kidney and hence attention to dosing may be needed in the critically ill patient.

Some commonly used antibiotics that are eliminated via the kidneys to a greater extent include:

- ampicillin
- cefuroxime
- erythromycin
- imipenem
- cephalosporins
- vancomycin
- nalidixic acid

73

Table 4.5   Some effects of antibiotics on renal function and their possible systemic sequelae to the patient.

	Type of renal damage	Hazards of excess accumulation
Aminoglycosides	RTN	Ototoxicity Further renal damage
Amphotericin B	RTN	
Nitrofurantoin	RTN	Peripheral neuropathy
Penicillins	Int. nephritis	Convulsions Haemolytic anaemia
Quinolones	RTO	
Sulphonamides	RTO Int. nephritis	
Tetracyclines	unknown	Nausea, vomiting, diarrhoea Dehydration Increased uraemia causing antianabolic effect
Vancomycin	Int. nephritis	Ototoxicity

RTN, renal tubular necrosis; RTO, renal tubular obstruction; Int. nephritis, interstitial nephritis

- benzylpenicillin
- co-trimoxazole
- gentamcin
- teicoplanin
- ethambutol
- nitrofurantoin
- metronidazole.

For co-trimoxazole, if the creatinine clearance is less than 20 ml/min, the dose should be reduced by 25%. For gentamicin, if the creatinine clearance is less than 50 ml/min, there should be a reduction in dose and an increase of the dosing interval.

The principles of safe therapy can be typified by considering the two drugs minocycline and cefazolin.[163,164] Minocycline is totally metabolised by the liver, and hence there is no relationship between creatinine clearance and half-life. By contrast, cefazolin is dependent on the kidney for its elimination, and exhibits a progressive and hyperbolic increase in its elimination half-life with the decrease in a patient's creatinine clearance. In the latter case, the impairment in creatinine clearance does not become clinically important until creatinine clearance is less than about 40 ml/min (Fig. 4.5). The latter is normally determined over a 24-hour period, but studies by Sladen et al. showed that in acutely ill patients, a two-hour creatinine clearance provides a useful index of changing renal function, and can be used to assess modifications in antibiotic and other drug dosage regimens.[165]

Thus, in all grades of renal failure, the doses of cephalosporins, ethambutol and vancomycin should be reduced; plasma concentrations of the

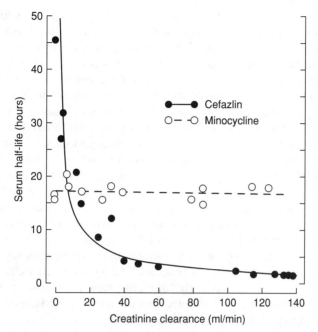

Figure 4.5   Relationship between creatinine clearance (ml/min) and serum half-lives of cefazolin and minocycline. (Redrawn[163,164])

aminoglycosides should be monitored daily to avoid ototoxicity and further renal damage; and drugs such as tetracyclines (with the exception of doxy-cycline), nitrofurantoin, and nalidixic acid are avoided. The doses of metronidazole, co-trimoxazole and the β-lactams will need modification. There have been a number of attempts made to relate the kinetics of drugs in renal failure to microbiological outcomes, with the development of nomograms. Typical examples are those for cefotaxime and ceftazi-dine,[166,167] although other authors have found them unreliable.[168]

Probably of greater importance is the influence of renal impairment on the disposition of the aminoglycosides (for example, gentamicin). The kinetics of these drugs show wide variability even in patients with normal renal function; for example Zaske *et al.* found an 80-fold variation in the elimination half-life and a 50-fold variation in daily dosage requirements to achieve therapeutic levels in surgical patients.[169] In order to facilitate achieving the desired efficacy of treatment by the aminoglycosides, Sawchuk *et al.* described in 1977 a method for calculating drug clearance and its volume of distribution based on a one-compartment model utilising three post-distributional plasma concentrations.[170] In a separate study which compared such a kinetically based dosing strategy with one using a nomogram relating the dose prescribed to the patient's creatinine clear-ance, Hickling *et al.* found higher peak and trough concentrations in the group where dosing was individually based on a two-hour creatinine clearance estimate taken from a nomogram when compared with those patients treated by doses of gentamicin or tobramycin as calculated according to the Sawchuk et al. model.[171] Based on the measurement of achieved drug concentrations, significantly fewer patients needed changes to their dosing strategy among those in the derived kinetic group (5 out of 13) compared with 11 out of 14 in the control group. The reasons for the changes were aminoglycoside concentrations at 48–72 hours outside the predetermined range for the peak or trough (suggesting that the initial dosing strategy was either too small or too large). These changes in drug dosing could not be attributed to any change in the routine indices of renal function monitored in the study. Although Mitchell et al. have shown that the volume of distribution of many aminoglycosides is increased by up to 40% in the critically ill,[172] most intensivists would not increase the loading dose of the antibiotic for the fear of causing systemic toxicity. More recently, Watling and Kisor have extended this approach by using population-derived pharmacokinetic modelling to develop a dosing nomogram for critically ill ICU patients.[173] This was based on the program NPEM (non-parametric expectation maximisation). Interestingly, the generated population parameter values were similar to those calculated by the Sawchuk–Zaske method, but had the advantage of improving the size of the initial dose such that therapeutic concentrations of the antibiotics were achieved earlier during treatment. Representative concentrations in the serum and peritoneal dialysate with some of the important antibiotics used in the critically ill patient are shown in Table 4.6.

Other complications to antibiotic dosing include the institution of venovenous and arteriovenous haemofiltration and haemodialysis. The main factors that influence drug removal by haemodialysis include molecular weight, lipid solubility, the extent of the drug's plasma protein binding and the efficiency of the dialyser. Thus water-soluble drugs with low molecular weights and small volumes of distribution are easily removed. However, extracorporeal clearance (EC Cl) as a means of drug elimination is really only relevant in clinical practice where the achieved EC Cl is >30% of total body clearance. Other determinants of extracorporeal drug removal relate to the membrane (and especially its permeability and binding characteristics) and the technique used (removal by haemofiltration depending on convection, and haemodialysis by diffusive principles). Using standard formulae, the clinician is able to calculate the expected extracorporeal clearances.

The theoretical basis of drug elimination through extracorporeal clearance by haemofiltration, haemodialysis, and haemodiafiltration is shown below:

$$Cl_{HF} = Q_F \times S\ (\alpha)$$
$$Cl_{HD} = Q_d \times S_d\ \{= C_d/C_p\}$$
$$Cl_{HDF} = [Q_F \times S\ (\alpha)] + [Q_d \times S_d]$$

Table 4.6   Serum concentrations and peritoneal dialysis fluid concentrations associated with therapeutic effects of some antimicrobials used in the ICU.

	Concentration (μg/ml)		
	Trough	Peak	Dialysate
Aminoglycosides			
Gentamicin	<2	4–8	4–8
Amikacin	<5	15–25	25
Netilmicin	<2	5–12	4–8
Tobramycin	<2.5	4–8	4–8
Streptomycin	<3	25	
Others			
Vancomycin	5–10	18–26	25
Teicoplanin	10–20	20–40	
Sulphamethoxazole	NR	200	
Fluconazole	15	25	
Flucytosine	NR	30–80	
Ciprofloxacin	1–2	3–5	
Chloramphenicol	5–10	25	
Ampicillin			125
Azlocillin			250
Cefuroxime			125
Ceftazidine			125

All peak levels should be taken one hour after the dose except for vancomycin (where the drug is given by infusion, and hence it should be two hours after starting the infusion), and chloramphenicol (two hours after the dose). The trough concentrations marked as NR are not relevant to therapeutic drug monitoring.

where HF is haemofiltration; HD is haemodialysis; HDF is haemodiafiltration; Q_F is ultrafiltration rate; S is sieving coefficient; Q_d is dialysate flow; C_d/C_p is dialysate saturation (= concentration in dialysate/concentration in plasma); α is unbound fraction of drug in the plasma, and S_d is dialysate saturation. Once the extent of extracorporeal clearance (Fr_{EC}) is known, then the dosage regimen can be adjusted such that:

$$I = I_{anuria} \times (1 - Fr_{EC})$$

and

$$D = \frac{D_{anuria}}{1 - Fr_{EC}}$$

where I_{anuria} is dosing interval and D_{anuria} is dose in anuric patients as quoted in the literature. The kinetic properties for drug removal by extracorporeal elimination are listed in Table 4.7. As already mentioned, for most drugs, the fractional extracorporeal clearance (expressed as a % of total body clearance) is low. However, examples of drugs that are significantly eliminated

77

Table 4.7   Physicochemical properties of drugs that can be effectively removed by haemodialysis or haemofiltration.

Haemodialysis	Haemofiltration
Relatively small molecular weight (MW) (<500)	MW less than the cut-off of the filter fibres (<40 000)
Water soluble	
Small volume of distribution (<1 l/kg)	Small volume of distribution (<1 l/kg)
Poorly protein bound	
Single-compartment kinetics	Single-compartment kinetics
Low endogenous clearance (<4 ml/kg/min)	Low endogenous clearance (<4 ml/kg/min)

from the body by a four-hour period of dialysis (and which are of interest to the intensivist) include:

- pentobarbitone
- monoamine oxidase inhibitors
- cimetidine
- ranitidine
- theophylline
- methylprednisolone
- mannitol
- aminophylline
- atenolol.

Other EC$_j$ methods of drug elimination include haemoperfusion, and drugs which would be removed to a significant extent by this means include pentobarbitone, cimetidine, aminophylline, theophylline, digoxin, quinidine, ampicillin, clindamycin, gentamicin and isoniazid. As a practical example of the effects of the institution of extracorporeal clearance on antibiotic disposition, the effects of venovenous haemofiltration on meziocillin kinetics were studied in eight patients with multi-organ failure and eight ICU patients without renal impairment.[174] In the filtration group, the half-life of the antibiotic was prolonged from 109 to 170 minutes. There was no absorption, however, of the antibiotic on to the filter membrane.

Antibiotic dosing in renal failure

If a drug has a high therapeutic ratio (as is the case with penicillins, cephalosporins, quinolones), appropriate dosing can usually be achieved by referral to strategies based on nomograms relating dose and creatinine clearance. However, for drugs with low therapeutic indices (for example, aminoglycosides and vancomycin) therapeutic drug monitoring is mandatory.

In general, penicillins have a low volume of distribution and variable plasma protein binding. Although they are eliminated through the kidney, dosage adjustments are rarely needed except for the penicillinase-resistant drugs that have a high renal clearance and high protein binding. Cephalosporins are significantly eliminated through the kidneys, and dosage adjustments are necessary in renal failure; however, significant extracorporeal elimination by haemodialysis or haemofiltration is only seen in patients being treated with cefuroxime, ceftazidine, and cefamandole.

Imipenem has a high non-renal clearance, but in some combinations with cilastatin the latter drug may accumulate, and is significantly cleared by extracorporeal elimination.

The β-lactamase inhibitors are not significantly eliminated by the various renal replacement therapies, as is also the case with the quinolones. However, both the aminoglycosides and the glycopeptides are significantly removed by extracorporeal methods, although there is also need for dosage reduction in cases of renal failure. Erythromycin, chloramphenicol, clindamycin, trimethoprim, metronidazole, and rifampicin are not removed by replacement therapy. For further details, the reader is referred to Schetz *et al*.[175] In general, if the ratio of free drug in plasma: volume of distribution (in l/kg) is >80, then haemodialysis will lead to the removal of a significant amount of drug (20–50%) in a six-hour dialysis; if the ratio is <20, then <10% of drug will be removed in the same time period.[176]

Use of inotropes and other cardiovascularly active drugs in the critically ill patient with renal impairment

Many of the drugs used to support the heart and circulation (for example, catecholamines and phosphodiesterase inhibitors) have short elimination half-lives and rapid dynamic responses and hence their effects are usually achieved by drug delivery by variable rate infusions. Because of their elimination half-lives of 2–3 minutes, stable blood concentrations are achieved within 10–15 minutes. Furthermore, the effects of the catecholamines appear to be linearly related to the blood concentration. Most are metabolised by the same pathways as the endogenous amines (neuronal uptake, monoamine oxidase, catechol-O-transferase).

There are no data in the literature on the effects of critical illness and renal impairment on the handling of adrenaline (epinephrine) and noradrenaline (norepinephrine).[177] Similarly, in the critically ill patient, dopamine has a transient dynamic effect and although there is considerable inter-patient variability in drug clearance (10–45 ml/kg/min), there is no obvious alteration in drug dynamics in the renally impaired subject.[178] Dopamine at low infusion rates (<2 μg/kg/min) predominantly stimulates the DA_1 receptor, which causes increased renal, mesenteric and coronary perfusion. This acts to increase urine output and drug excretion in the normovolaemic patient. At higher infusion rates (2–5 μg/kg/min), dopamine shows dose-dependent β_1-(and to a lesser extent β_2) effects, while the α-effects are predominant at rates >5 μg/kg/min. The dopaminergic effect is through an inhibition of Na^+/K^+ ATPase activity, which leads to increased urinary sodium excretion. These effects are blocked by dopamine antagonists such as phenothiazines, butyrophenones, and metoclopramide.

Dobutamine has a predominant β_1 action, leading to an increase in cardiac output. The drug is made up of two isomers: the l form is mainly an α-agonist, while the d form is a β_1-agonist. These isomers cancel each other out *in vivo* such that the drug has little effect on peripheral vascular beds. The clearance of dobutamine is also high (53–59 ml/kg/min).

Dopexamine (a new synthetic agent) is mainly a β_2-agonist, with weak agonist properties on the DA_1, DA_2 and β_1 receptors. The amine has no α-agonist effects. It acts to improve tissue perfusion by splanchnic vasodilatation such that there are decreases in systemic and pulmonary artery pressures. The renal effects of dopexamine are by renal tubular DA_1 stimulation as well as renal vasodilatation, so increasing sodium excretion, the creatinine clearance, glomerular filtration rate, and urinary volume. Thus it will be expected to increase renal drug elimination.

However, there is a further complicating factor to dosing by the catecholamines in that there may occur a change in receptor responsiveness (up- and down-regulation). The latter is often seen in the critically ill patient, and results in increased drug requirements which are dynamic and not kinetic in origin.

Another drug that increases renal blood flow (and hence potentially drug elimination) is fenoldopam (a benzodiazepine derivative) which is a selective DA_1-agonist, causing peripheral vasodilatation and decreases in blood pressure. Again, it causes an increased glomerular filtration rate and hence urinary drug excretion.

Another important inotrope is digoxin, whose half-life in the patient with normal renal function is about 1·6 days; this may increase significantly to over 100 hours in patients with renal dysfunction. Under such circumstances, the maintenance dose of digoxin may need to be only 33% of that in healthy patients.[179] Hence the maintenance dose of digoxin should be reduced from the usual dose range of 125–500 µg to one that is only one-third to one-half that used in patients with normal renal function. Digoxin is also significantly removed from the body by high-performance renal replacement therapies. Furthermore, its clearance may also be decreased by the concomitant administration of other cardioactive drugs such as verapamil, quinidine, amiodarone, propafenone, diltiazem, and nicardipine.[180] Digoxin toxicity can also arise in the critically ill patient by the associated development of hypokalaemia or hypomagnesaemia through treatment with drugs such as amphotericin B, β_2-mimetics, corticosteroids, and loop and thiazide diuretics. The situation is further complicated by the non-reliability of assays for plasma digoxin concentrations in the critically ill patients. Many of the immunoassays show cross-reactivity with metabolites of digoxin as well as with digoxin-like substances which accumulate in some patients with renal failure.[181]

Similarly, steroids, insulin, anticoagulants, thrombolytic agents, anti-hypertensive drugs, and nitrates are usually dosed according to their effect; however, sodium nitroprusside should probably not be continued for more than two days in patients with renal impairment because some of its metabolites (for example, cyanide) may be toxic.

Other drugs often administered to critically ill patients include the H_2-receptor antagonists where there is a need to reduce the dose by about 20–50% in patients with renal failure, but there is no significant further effect of renal replacement therapy. The clinician should avoid giving aluminium, magnesium, and bismuth antacids to patients with renal failure, as these may accumulate and toxicity develop. However, sucralfate (a non-absorbable aluminium salt of sucrose octasulphate) appears to be safe to use in the critically ill patient with renal dysfunction. The antiemetics metoclopramide and prochlorperazine should be given in reduced doses, otherwise the side effects of dystonia and cerebral stimulation, respectively, may occur.

Loop diuretics can be effectively administered at increased doses in the critically ill patient with renal failure and fluid overload, although dosing is best based on titration according to response. However, in patients with renal impairment, other diuretics such as frusemide and bumetanide will normally only produce a response in very high doses, although there is the potential problem of ototoxicity especially with the latter agent. Antihypertensive agents (such as hydralazine, labetalol, and nifedipine) all show increased pharmacological effects in the patient with renal failure, and hence lower than usual doses should be given (at least initially). The use of potassium-sparing diuretics is generally contraindicated in the critically ill patient with renal failure

Thus the intensivist, with a wide range of drug choices, should be cautious of the altered effects that may occur when they are administered to the critically ill patient with renal failure. There are few drugs where there is no alteration in their kinetics or dynamics, or where drug–drug interactions may not occur. Only by vigilance and the careful reporting of adverse side effects can we be sure of rational and safe treatment in this group of patients.

1 Verbeeck RK, Branch RA, Wilkinson GR. Drug metabolites in renal failure: pharmacokinetic and clinical implications. *Clin Pharmacokinet* 1981;6:329–45.
2 Terner UK, Wiebe LI, Noujain AA, Dossetor JB, Sanders EJ. The effects of acute and chronic uremia in rats on their hepatic microsomal enzyme activity. *Clin Biochem* 1978;11:156–8.
3 Rice SA, Sievenpiper TS, Mazze RI. Liver function and anesthetic metabolism in rats with chronic renal impairment. *Anesthesiology* 1984;60:418–21.
4 Dundee JW, Richards RK. Effect of azotemia upon the action of barbiturate anesthesia. *Anesthesiology* 1954;13:333–46.
5 Freeman BB, Sheff MF, Maher JF, Schreiner GE. The blood–cerebrospinal fluid barrier in uremia. *Ann Intern Med* 1962;56:233–40.
6 Burch PG, Stanski DR. Decreased protein binding and thiopental kinetics. *Clin Pharmacol Ther* 1982;32:212–17.
7 Christensen JH, Andreasen F, Jansen J. Pharmacokinetics and pharmacodynamics of thiopental in patients undergoing renal transplantation. *Acta Anaesthesiol Scand* 1983;27:513–18.
8 Shoeman DW, Azarnoff DL. The alterations of plasma proteins in uremia as reflected by their ability to bind digitoxin and diphenylhydratoin. *Pharmacology* 1972;7:169–77.
9 Richet G, de Novales EL, Verroust P. Drug intoxication and neurological episodes in chronic renal failure. *Br Med J* 1970;ii:394–5.
10 Reidenberg MM, Lowenthal DT, Briggs W, Gasparo M. Pentobarbital elimination in patients with poor renal function. *Clin Pharmacol Ther* 1976;20:67–71.

11 Vinik HR, Reves JG, Greenblatt DJ, Abernethy DR, Smith LR. The pharmacokinetics of midazolam in chronic renal failure patients. *Anesthesiology* 1983;**59**:390–4.

12 Ochs HR, Greenblatt DJ, Kaschel HJ, Kleht W, Divoll M, Abernethy DR. Diazepam kinetics in patients with renal insufficiency or hyperthyroidism. *Br J Clin Pharmacol* 1981;**12**:829–32.

13 Carlos R, Calvo R, Erill S. Plasma protein binding of etomidate in patients with renal failure or hepatic cirrhosis. *Clin Pharmacokinet* 1979;**4**:144–8.

14 Kirvela M, Olkkola KT, Rosenberg PH, Yli-Hankala A, Salmela K, Lindgren L. Pharmacokinetics of propofol and haemodynamic changes during induction of anaesthesia in uraemic patients. *Br J Anaesth* 1992;**68**:178–82.

15 Costela JL, Jimenez R, Calvo R, Suarez E, Carlos R. Serum protein binding of propofol in patients with renal failure or hepatic cirrhosis. *Acta Anaesthesiol Scand* 1996;**40**:741–5.

16 Ickx B, Cockshott ID, Barvais L *et al*. Propofol infusion for induction and maintenance of anaesthesia in patients with end-stage renal disease. *Br J Anaesth* 1998;**81**:854–60.

17 Albanese J, Martin C, Lacarelle B, Saux P, Durand A, Gouin F. Pharmackinetics of long-term propofol infusion used for sedation in ICU patients. *Anesthesiology* 1990;**73**:214–17.

18 Bailie GR, Cockshott ID, Douglas EJ, Bowles BJM. Pharmacokinetics of propofol during and after long term continuous infusion for maintenance of sedation in ICU patients. *Br J Anaesth* 1992;**86**:486–91.

19 Snellen F, Lauwers P, Demeyere R, Byttebier G, Van Aken H. The use of midazolam versus propofol for short-term sedation following coronary artery bypass grafting. *Intens Care Med* 1990;**16**:312–16.

20 Beller JP, Pottecher T, Lugnier A, Mangin P, Otteni JC. Prolonged sedation with propofol in ICU patients: recovery and blood concentration changes during periodic interruptions in infusion. *Br J Anaesth* 1988;**61**:583–8.

21 Eddleston JM, Pollard BJ, Blades JF, Doran B. The use of propofol for sedation of critically ill patients undergoing haemodiafiltration. *Intens Care Med* 1995;**21**:342–7.

22 Shafer A, Doze VA, White PF. Pharmacokinetic variability of midazolam infusions in critically ill patients. *Crit Care Med* 1990;**18**:1039–41.

23 Oldenhof H, de Jong M, Steenhoek A, Janknegt R. Clinical pharmacokinetics of midazolam in intensive care patients, a wide interpatient variability? *Clin Pharmacol Ther* 1988;**43**:263–9.

24 Bauer TM, Ritz R, Haberthur C *et al*. Prolonged sedation due to accumulation of conjugated metabolites of midazolam. *Lancet* 1995;**346**:145–7.

25 Shelly MP, Sultan MA, Bodenham A, Park GR. Midazolam infusions in critically ill patients. *Eur J Anaesthesiol* 1991;**8**:21–7.

26 Kangas L, Kanto J, Forsstrom J, Ilisalo E. The protein binding of diazepam and N-desmethyldiazepam in patients with poor renal function. *Clin Nephrol* 1976;**5**:114–18.

27 Verbeeck R, Tjandramanga TB, Verberckmoes R, de Schepper PJ. Biotransformation and excretion of lorazepam in patients with chronic renal failure. *Br J Clin Pharmacol* 1976;**3**:1033–39.

28 Verbeeck RV, Tjandramanga TB, Verberckmoes R, de Schepper PJ. Impaired elimination of lorazepam following subchronic administration in two patients with renal failure. *Br J Clin Pharmacol* 1981;**12**:749–51.

29 Hanna MH, Peat SJ, Woodham M, Knibb A, Fung C. Analgesic efficacy and CSF pharmacokinetics of intrathecal morphine-6-glucuronide: comparison with morphine. *Br J Anaesth* 1990;**64**:547–50.

30 Smith MT, Watt JA, Cramond T. Morphine-3-glucuronide: a potent antagonist of morphine analgesia. *Life Sci* 1990;**47**:579–85.

31 Watt JA, Cramond T, Smith MT. Morphine-6-glucuronide: analgesic effects antagonised by morphine-3-glucuronide. *Clin Exp Pharmacol Physiol* 1990;**17**:83(abstract).

32 Mostert JW, Evers JL, Hobika GH, Moore RH, Ambrus JL. Cardiorespiratory effects of anaesthesia with morphine or fentanyl in chronic renal failure and cerebral toxicity after morphine. *Br J Anaesth* 1971;**43**:1053–9.

33 Don HF, Dieppa RA, Taylor P. Narcotic analgesics in anuric patients. *Anesthesiology* 1975;**42**:745–7.

34 Stanley TH, Lathrop GD. Urinary excretion of morphine during and after valvular and coronary-artery surgery. *Anesthesiology* 1977;**46**:166–9.

35 Olsen GD, Bennett WM, Porter GA. Morphine and phenytoin binding to plasma proteins in renal and hepatic failure. *Clin Pharmacol Ther* 1975;**17**:677–84.

82

36 Sloan PA, Mather LE, McLean CF *et al*. Physiological disposition of i.v. morphine in sheep. *Br J Anaesth* 1991;**67**:378–86.
37 Milne RW, Sloan PA, McLean CF *et al*. The disposition of morphine and its 3- and 6-glucuronide metabolites during morphine infusion in the sheep. *Drug Metab Dispos* 1993;**21**:1151–6.
38 Milne RW, McLean CF, Mather LE *et al*. Comparative disposition of morphine-3-glucuronide during separate intravenous infusions of morphine and morphine-3-glucuronide in sheep. Importance of the kidney. *Drug Metab Dispos* 1995;**23**: 334–42.
39 Milne RE, McLean CF, Mather LE *et al*. Influence of renal failure on the disposition of morphine, morphine-3-glucuronide and morphine-6-glucuronide in sheep during intravenous infusion with morphine. *J Pharmacol Exp Ther* 1997;**282**:779–86.
40 Sear JW, Hand CW, Moore RA, McQuay HJ. Studies on morphine disposition: influence of renal failure renal on the kinetics of morphine and its metabolites. *Br J Anaesth* 1989;**62**:28–32.
41 Aitkenhead AR, Vater M, Achola K, Cooper CMS, Smith G. Pharmacokinetics of single-dose iv morphine in normal volunteers and patients with end-stage renal failure. *Br J Anaesth* 1984;**56**:813–18.
42 Sawe J, Odar-Cederlof I. Kinetics of morphine in patients with renal failure. *Eur J Clin Pharmacol* 1987;**32**:337–42.
43 Woolner DF, Winter D, Frendin TJ, Begg EJ, Linn KL, Wright GJ. Renal failure does not impair the metabolism of morphine. *Br J Clin Pharmacol* 1986;**22**:55–9.
44 Chauvin M, Sandouk P, Scherrmann JM, Farinotti R, Strumza P, Duvaldestin P. Morphine pharmacokinetics in renal failure. *Anesthesiology* 1987;**66**:327–31.
45 Osborne R, Joel S, Grebenik K, Trew D, Slevin K. The pharmacokinetics of morphine and morphine glucuronides in kidney failure. *Clin Pharmacol Ther* 1993;**54**:158–67.
46 Mazoit JX, Sandouk P, Scherrmann J-M, Roche A. Extrahepatic metabolism of morphine occurs in humans. *Clin Pharmacol Ther* 1990;**48**:613–18.
47 Milne RW, Nation RL, Somogyi AA, Bochner F, Griggs WM. The influence of renal function on the renal clearance of morphine and its glucuronide metabolites in intensive-care patients. *Br J Clin Pharmacol* 1992;**34**:53–9.
48 Petersen GM, Randall CTC, Paterson J. Plasma levels of morphine and morphine glucuronides in the treatment of cancer pain: relationship to renal function and route of administration. *Eur J Clin Pharmacol* 1990;**38**:121–4.
49 Loetsch J, Stockmann A, Kobal G *et al*. Pharmacokinetics of morphine and its glucuronides after intravenous infusion of morphine and morphine-6-glucuronide in healthy volunteers. *Clin Pharmacol Ther* 1996;**60**:316–25.
50 Osborne RJ, Joel SP, Slevin ML. Morphine intoxication in renal failure: the role of morphine-6-glucuronide. *Br Med J* 1986;**292**:1548–9.
51 Shelly MP, Cory EP, Park GR. Pharmacokinetics of morphine in two children before and after liver transplantation. *Br J Anaesth* 1986;**58**:1218–23.
52 Hasselstrom J, Berg U, Lofgren A, Sawe J. Long lasting respiratory depression induced by morphine-6-glucuronide? *Br J Clin Pharmacol* 1989;**27**:515–18.
53 Covington EC, Gonsalves-Ebrahim L, Currie KO, Shepard KV, Pippenger CE. Severe respiratory depression from patient-controlled analgesia in renal failure. *Psychosomatics* 1989;**30**:226–8.
54 Carr AC, Stone PA, Serpell MG, Joel SP, Tinker L. Patient controlled morphine analgesia (PCA morphine) in cadaveric renal transplant recipients: does morphine-6-glucuronide accumulate? *Br J Anaesth* 1998;**81**:630p (abstract).
55 D'Honneur G, Gilton A, Sandouk P, Scherrmann JM, Duvaldestin P. Plasma and cerebrospinal fluid concentrations of morphine and morphine glucuronides after oral morphine. The influence of renal failure. *Anesthesiology* 1994;**81**:87–93.
56 Carrupt PA, Testa B, Bechalany A, el-Tayar N, Descas P, Perrissoud D. Morphine 6-glucuronide and morphine 3-glucuronide as molecular chameleons with unexpected lipophilicity. *J Med Chem* 1991;**34**:1272–5.
57 Portenoy RK, Thaler HT, Inturrisi CE, Friedlanderklar H, Foley KM. The metabolite morphine-6-glucuronide contributes to the analgesia produced by morphine infusion in patients with pain and normal renal function. *Clin Pharmacol Ther* 1992;**51**:422–31.
58 Faura CC, Collins SL, Moore RA, McQuay HJ. Systematic review of factors affecting the ratios of morphine and its major metabolites. *Pain* 1998;**74**:43–53.
59 Bion JF, Logan BK, Newman PM *et al*. Sedation in intensive care: morphine and renal function. *Intens Care Med* 1986;**12**:359–65.

60 Davies JG, Combes ID, Kingswood C, Ruprah M, Street M. The clearance of morphine and morphine-6-glucuronide in critically ill patients receiving continuous renal replacement therapies (abstract). *J Pharm Pharmacol* 1994;**46** (suppl 2): 1045.

61 Glare PA, Walsh TD, Pippenger CE. Normorphine, a neurotoxic metabolite? *Lancet* 1990;**335**:725–6.

62 Gibson TP, Giacomini KM, Briggs WA, Whitman W, Levy G. Propoxyphene and norpropoxyphene plasma concentrations in the anephric patient. *Clin Pharmacol Ther* 1980;**27**:665–70.

63 Barnes JN, Williams AJ, Tomson MJF, Toseland PA, Goodwin FJ. Dihydrocodeine in renal failure: further evidence for an important role of the kidney in the handling of opioid drugs. *BMJ* 1985;**290**:740–2.

64 Guay DRP, Awni WM, Findlay JWA *et al*. Pharmacokinetics and pharmacodynamics of codeine in end-stage renal disease. *Clin Pharmacol Ther* 1988;**43**:63–71.

65 Fishman RA. Permeability changes in experimental uremic encephalopathy. *Arch Intern Med* 1970;**126**:835–7.

66 Lowenthal DT. Tissue sensitivity to drugs in disease states. *Med Clin North Am* 1974;**58**:1111–19.

67 Corall IM, Moore AR, Strunin L. Plasma concentrations of fentanyl in normal surgical patients and those with severe renal and hepatic disease. *Br J Anaesth* 1980;**52**:101p.

68 Sear JW. Disposition of fentanyl and alfentanil in patients undergoing renal transplantation. In Bergmann H, Steinbereithner K, eds. VII European Congress of Anaesthesiology, Proceedings I (main topics 1–6) *Beitr Anaesthesiol Intensivmed* 1987;**19**:53–8.

69 Koren G, Crean P, Goresky GV, Klein J, MacLeod SM. Pharmacokinetics of fentanyl in children with renal disease. *Res Commun Chem Pathol Pharmacol* 1984;**46**:371–9.

70 Duthie DJR. Renal failure, surgery and fentanyl pharmacokinetics. In Bergmann H, Steinbereithner K, eds. Proceedings of VII European Congress of Anaesthesiology, volume II. *Beitr Anaesthesiol Intensivmed* 1987;**20**:374–5.

71 Koehntop DE, Rodman JH. Fentanyl pharmacokinetics in patients undergoing renal transplantation. *Pharmacotherapy* 1997;**17**:746–52.

72 Bower S. Plasma protein binding of fentanyl: the effect of hyperlipidaemia and chronic renal failure. *J Pharm Pharmacol* 1982;**34**:102–6.

73 Alazia M, Levron JC. Etude pharmacocinétique d'une perfusion intraveineuse prolongée de fentanyl en réanimation. *Ann Fr Anesth Reanim* 1987;**6**:465–6.

74 Chauvin M, Lebrault C, Levron JC, Duvaldestin P. Pharmacokinetics of alfentanil in chronic renal failure. *Anesth Analg* 1987;**66**:53–6.

75 Bower S, Sear JW. Disposition of alfentanil in patients receiving a renal transplant. *J Pharm Pharmacol* 1989;**41**:654–7.

76 Kharasch ED, Russell M, Mautz D *et al*. The role of cytochrome P450 3A4 in alfentanil clearance. Implications for interindividual variability in disposition and perioperative drug interactions. *Anesthesiology* 1997;**87**:36–50.

77 Koehntop DE, Noormohamed SE, Fletcher CV. Effects of long-term drugs on alfentanil clearance in patients undergoing renal transplantation. *Pharmacotherapy* 1994;**14**:592–9.

78 Sinclair ME, Sear JW, Summerfield RJ, Fisher A. Alfentanil infusions on the Intensive Therapy Unit. *Intens Care Med* 1988;**14**:55–9.

79 Fyman PN, Reynolds JR, Moser F, Avitable M, Casthely PA, Butt K. Pharmacokinetics of sufentanil in patients undergoing renal transplantation. *Can J Anaesth* 1988;**35**:312–15.

80 Davis PJ, Stiller RL, Cook DR, Brandom BW, Davin-Robinson KA. Pharmacokinetics of sufentanil in adolescent patients with chronic renal failure. *Anesth Analg* 1988;**67**:268–71.

81 Sear JW. Sufentanil disposition in patients undergoing renal transplantation: influence of choice of kinetic model. *Br J Anaesth* 1989;**63**:60–7.

82 Wiggum DC, Cork RC, Weldon ST, Gandolfi AJ, Perry DS. Postoperative respiratory depression and elevated sufentanil levels in a patient with chronic renal failure. *Anesthesiology* 1985;**63**:708–10.

83 Hoke FJ, Shlugman D, Dershwitz M *et al*. Pharmacokinetics and pharmacodynamics of remifentanil in persons with renal failure compared with healthy volunteers. *Anesthesiology* 1997;**87**:533–41.

84 Kirvela M, Lindgren L, Seppala T, Olkkola KT. The pharmacokinetics of oxycodone in uremic patients undergoing renal transplantation. *J Clin Anesth* 1996;**8**:13–18.

85 Mather LE, Tucker GT, Pflug AE, Lindop MJ, Wilkerson C. Meperidine kinetics in man. Intravenous injection in surgical patients and volunteers. *Clin Pharmacol Ther* 1975;**17**:21–30.

86 Edwards DJ, Svensson CK, Visco JP, Lalka D. Clinical pharmacokinetics of pethidine. *Clin Pharmacokinet* 1982;**7**:421–33.

87 Chan K, Tse J, Jenning F, Orme ML. Pharmacokinetics of low-dose intravenous pethidine in patients with renal dysfunction. *J Clin Pharmacol* 1987;**27**:516–22.

88 Burgess KR, Burgess EE, Whitelaw WA. Impaired ventilatory response to carbon dioxide in patients in chronic renal failure: implications for the intensive care unit. *Crit Care Med* 1994;**22**:413–19.

89 Szeto HH, Inturrisi CE, Houde R, Saal S, Cheigh J, Reidenberg M. Accumulation of normeperidine, an active metabolite of meperidine in patients with renal failure or cancer. *Ann Intern Med* 1977;**86**:738–41.

90 Odar-Cederlof I, Boreus LO, Bondesson U, Holmberg L, Heyner L. Comparison of renal excretion of pethidine (meperidine) and its metabolites in old and young patients. *Eur J Clin Pharmacol* 1985;**28**:171–5.

91 Mather LE, Meffin PJ. Clinical pharmacokinetics of pethidine. *Clin Pharmacokinet* 1978;**3**:352–68.

92 Armstrong PJ, Bersten A. Normeperidine toxicity. *Anesth Analg* 1986;**65**:536–8.

93 Turner SA, Denson DD, Sollo D, Katz J. Extraction of narcotics by hemodialysis. *Reg Anesth* 1990;**15** (suppl):14 (abstract).

94 Hand CW, Sear JW, Uppington J, Ball MJ, McQuay HJ, Moore RA. Buprenorphine disposition in patients with renal impairment: single and continuous dosing with especial reference to metabolites. *Br J Anaesth* 1990;**64**:276–82.

95 Levine DF. Hypocalcaemia increases the narcotic effect of codeine. *Postgrad Med J* 1980;**56**:736–7.

96 Matzke GR, Chan GLC, Abrahim PA. Codeine dosage in renal failure. *Clin Pharmacol* 1986;**5**:15–16.

97 Redfern N. Dihydrocodeine overdose treated with naloxone infusion. *Br Med J* 1983;**287**:751–2.

98 Duthie DJR, Stevens JJWM, Doyle AR, Baddoo HHK. Remifentanil and coronary artery surgery. *Lancet* 1997;**345**:649–50.

99 Bacon R, Chandrasekan V, Haigh A, Royston BD, Royston D, Sundt T. Early extubation after open-heart surgery with total intravenous anaesthetic technique. *Lancet* 1995;**345**:133–4.

100 Shapiro BA, Warren J, Egol AB *et al.* Practice parameters for intravenous analgesia and sedation fot adult patients in the intensive care unit: an executive summary. *Crit Care Med* 1995;**23**:1596–600.

101 Wyant GM. The anaesthetist looks at tissue transplantation: three years' experience with kidney transplants. *Can Anaesth Soc J* 1967;**14**:255–75.

102 Way WL, Miller RD, Hamilton WK, Layzer RB. Succinylcholine-induced hyperkalemia in patients with renal failure? *Anesthesiology* 1972;**36**:138–41.

103 Gibaldi M, Levy G, Hayton EL. Tubocurarine and renal failure. *Br J Anaesth* 1972;**44**:163–5.

104 Matteo RS, Spector S, Horowitz PE. Relation of serum *d*-tubocurarine concentration to neuromuscular blockade in man. *Anesthesiology* 1974;**41**:440–3.

105 Miller RD, Matteo RS, Benet LZ, Sohn TI. The pharmacokinetics of *d*-tubocurarine in man with and without renal failure. *J Pharmacol Exp Ther* 1977;**202**:1–7.

106 Brotherton WD, Matteo RS. Pharmacokinetics and pharmacodynamics of metocurine in humans with and without renal failure. *Anesthesiology* 1981;**55**:273–6.

107 Ramzan MI, Shanks CA, Triggs EJ. Gallamine disposition in surgical patients with chronic renal failure. *Br J Clin Pharmacol* 1981;**12**:141–7.

108 McLeod K, Watson MJ, Rawlins MD. Pharmacokinetics of pancuronium in patients with normal and impaired renal function. *Br J Anaesth* 1976;**48**:341–5.

109 Somogyi AA, Shanks CA, Triggs EJ. The effect of renal failure on the disposition and neuromuscular blocking action of pancuronium bromide. *Eur J Clin Pharmacol* 1977;**12**:23–9.

110 Fahey MR, Rupp SM, Fisher DM *et al.* The pharmacokinetics and pharmacodynamics of atracurium in patients with and without renal failure. *Anesthesiology* 1984;**61**:699–702.

111 deBros FM, Lai A, Scott R *et al.* Pharmacokinetics and pharmacodynamics of atracurium during isoflurane anesthesia in normal and anephric patients. *Anesth Analg* 1986;**65**:743–6.

112 Eastwood NB, Boyd AH, Parker CJH, Hunter JM. Pharmacokinetics of 1R-*cis* 1R'-*cis* atracurium besylate (51W89) and plasma laudanosine concentrations in health and chronic renal failure. *Br J Anaesth* 1995;**75**:431–5.

113 Lynam DP, Cronnelly R, Castagnoli KP *et al*. The pharmacodynamics and pharmacokinetics of vecuronium in patients anesthetized with isoflurane with normal renal function or with renal failure. *Anesthesiology* 1988;**69**:227–31.

114 Head-Rapson AG, Devlin JC, Parker CJ, Hunter JM. Pharmacokinetics and pharmacodynamics of the three isomers of mivacurium in health, in end-stage renal failure and in patients with impaired renal function. *Br J Anaesth* 1995;**75**:31–6.

115 Szenohradszky J, Caldwell JE, Wright PMC *et al*. Influence of renal failure on the pharmacokinetics and neuromuscular blocking effects of a single dose of rapacuronium bromide. *Anesthesiology* 1999;**90**:24–35.

116 Caldwell JE, Canfell PC, Castagnoli KP *et al*. The influence of renal failure on the pharmacokinetics and duration of action of pipecuronium bromide in patients anesthetized with halothane and nitrous oxide. *Anesthesiology* 1989;**70**:7–12.

117 Cook DR, Freeman JA, Lai AA *et al*. Pharmacokinetics and pharmacodynamics of doxacurium in normal patients and in those with hepatic or renal failure. *Anesth Analg* 1991;**72**:145–50.

118 Szenohradszky J, Fisher DM, Segredo V *et al*. Pharmacokinetics of rocuronium bromide (ORG 9426) in patients with normal renal function or patients undergoing cadaver renal transplantation. *Anesthesiology* 1992;**77**:899–904.

119 Mushin WW, Wien R, Mason DFJ, Langston GT. Curare-like actions of tri-(diethylaminoethoxy)-benzene triethyliodide. *Lancet* 1949;**i**:726–8.

120 Feldman SA, Cohen EN, Golling RC. The excretion of gallamine in the dog. *Anesthesiology* 1969;**30**:593–8.

121 Buzello W, Agoston S. Pharmacokinetics of pancuronium in patients with normal and impaired renal function. *Anaesthesist* 1978;**27**:291–7.

122 Geha DG, Blitt CD, Moon BJ. Prolonged neuromuscular blockade with pancuronium in the presence of acute renal failure: a case report. *Anesth Analg* 1976;**55**:343–5.

123 Hunter JM, Jones RS, Utting JE. Use of atracurium in patients with no renal function. *Br J Anaesth* 1982;**54**:1251–8.

124 Hunter JM, Jones RS, Utting JE. Comparison of vecuronium, atracurium and tubocurarine in normal patients and in patients with no renal function. *Br J Anaesth* 1984;**56**:941–51.

125 Russo R, Ravagnan R, Buzzetti V, Favini P. Atracurium in patients with chronic renal failure. *Br J Anaesth* 1986;**58**(suppl 1):63s.

126 Richard JP, Conil JP, Antonini A, Bareille P. Utilisation du bromure de vecuronium administré a debit constant lors des transplantations rénales. *Cah Anesthesiol* 1986;**34**:125–6.

127 Nguyen HD, Kaplan R, Nagashima H, Dunclaf D, Foldes FF. The neuromuscular effect of atracurium in anephric patients. *Anesthesiology* 1985;**63**:A335.

128 Fisher DM, Canfell C, Fahey MR *et al*. Elimination of atracurium in humans: contribution of Hofmann elimination and ester hydrolysis versus organ-bound elimination. *Anesthesiology* 1986;**65**:6–12.

129 Yate PM, Flynn PJ, Arnold RW. Clinical experience and plasma laudanosine concentrations during the infusion of atracurium in the intensive therapy unit. *Br J Anaesth* 1987;**59**:211–17.

130 Ward S, Boheimer N, Weatherley BC, Simmonds RJ, Dopson TA. Pharmacokinetics of atracurium and its metabolites in patients with normal renal function, and in patients in renal failure. *Br J Anaesth* 1987;**59**:697–706.

131 Parker CJR, Jones JE, Hunter JM. Disposition of infusions of atracurium and its metabolite laudanosine in patients with renal and respiratory failure in an ITU. *Br J Anaesth* 1988;**61**:531–40.

132 Chapple DJ, Miller AA, Ward JB, Wheatley PL. Cardiovascular and neurological effects of laudanosine. Studies in mice and rats, and in conscious and anaesthetized dogs. *Br J Anaesth* 1987;**59**:218–25.

133 Fahey MR, Morris RB, Miller RD, Nguyen TL, Upton RA. Pharmacokinetics of ORG NC45 (Norcuron) in patients with and without renal failure. *Br J Anaesth* 1981;**53**:1049–53.

134 Shearer ES, O'Sullivan EP, Hunter JM. Clearance of atracurium and laudanosine in the urine and by continuous venovenous haemofiltration. *Br J Anaesth* 1991;**67**:569–73.

135 Hunter JM. Atracurium and laudanosine pharmacokinetics in acute renal failure. *Intens Care Med* 1993;**19**(suppl 2):s91–s93.

136 Bevan DR, Donati F, Gyasi H, Williams A. Vecuronium in renal failure. *Can Anaesth Soc J* 1984;**31**:491–6.

137 LePage JY, Malinge M, Cozian A, Pinaud M, Blanloeil Y, Souron R. Vecuronium and atracurium in patients with endstage renal failure. *Br J Anaesth* 1987;**59**:1004–10.

138 Cody MW, Dormon FM. Recurarisation after vecuronium in a patient with renal failure. *Anaesthesia* 1987;**42**:993–5.

139 Starsnic MA, Goldberg ME, Ritter DE, Marr AT, Sosis M, Larijani GE. Does vecuronium accumulate in the renal transplant patient? *Can J Anaesth* 1989;**36**:35–9.

140 Beauvoir C, Peray P, Daures JP, Peschaud JL, D'Athis F. Pharmacodynamics of vecuronium in patients with and without renal failure: a meta-analysis. *Can J Anaesth* 1993;**40**:696–702.

141 Smith CL, Hunter JM, Jones RS. Vecuronium infusions in patients with renal failure in an ITU. *Anaesthesia* 1987;**42**:387–93.

142 Segredo V, Caldwell JE, Matthay MA, Sharma ML, Gruenke LD, Miller RD. Persistent paralysis in critically ill patients after long-term administration of vecuronium. *New Engl J Med* 1992;**327**:524–8.

143 Lagasse RS, Katz RI, Petersen M, Jacobson MJ, Poppers PJ. Prolonged neuromuscular blockade following vecuronium infusion. *J Clin Anesth* 1990;**2**:269–71.

144 Caldwell JE, Szenohradszky J, Segredo V *et al.* The pharmacodynamics and pharmacokinetics of the metabolite 3-des-acetylvecuronium (Org 7268) and its parent compound, vecuronium, in human volunteers. *J Pharmacol Exp Ther* 1994;**270**: 1216–22.

145 Segredo V, Caldwell JE, Wright PMC, Sharma ML, Gruenke LD, Miller RD. Do the pharmacokinetics of vecuronium change during prolonged administration in the critically ill patients? *Br J Anaesth* 1998;**80**:715–19.

146 de Bros F, Basta SJ, Ali HH, Wargin W, Welch R. Pharmacokinetics and pharmacodynamics of BW B1090U in healthy surgical patients receiving N_2O/O_2 isoflurane anesthesia. *Anesthesiology* 1987;**67**:A609.

147 Cook DR, Freeman JA, Lai AA *et al.* Pharmacokinetics of mivacurium in normal patients and in those with hepatic or renal failure. *Br J Anaesth* 1992;**69**:580–5.

148 Phillips BJ, Hunter JM. Use of mivacurium chloride by constant infusion in the anephric patient. *Br J Anaesth* 1992;**68**:492–8.

149 Cashman JN, Luke JJ, Jones RM. Neuromuscular block with doxacurium (BW A938U) in patients with normal or absent renal function. *Br J Anaesth* 1992;**64**:186–92.

150 Murray MJ, Coursin DB, Scuderi PE *et al.* Double-blind, randomized, multicenter study of doxacurium vs. pancuronium in intensive care unit patients who require neuromuscular-blocking agents. *Crit Care Med* 1995;**23**:450–8.

151 Khuenl-Brady KS, Pomaroli A, Puhringer F, Mitterschiffthaler G, Koller J. The use of rocuronium (ORG 9426) in patients with chronic renal failure. *Anaesthesia* 1993;**48**:873–5.

152 Cooper RA, Maddineni VR, Mirakhur RK, Wierda JM, Brady M, Fitzpatrick KT. Time course of neuromuscular effects and pharmacokinetics of rocuronium bromide (Org 9426) during isoflurane anaesthesia in patients with and without renal failure. *Br J Anaesth* 1993;**71**:222–6.

153 Sparr HJ, Wierda JMKH, Proost JH, Keller C, Khuenl-Brady KS. Pharmacodynamics and pharmacokinetics of rocuronium in intensive care patients. *Br J Anaesth* 1997;**78**:267–73.

154 Kisor DF, Schmith VD, Wargin WA, Lien CA, Ornstein E, Cook DR. Importance of the organ-independent elimination of cisatracurium. *Anesth Analg* 1996;**83**:901–3.

155 Boyd AH, Eastwood NB, Parker CJH, Hunter JM. Pharmacodynamics of the 1R-*cis* 1R'-*cis* isomers of atracurium (51W89) in health and chronic renal failure. *Br J Anaesth* 1995;**74**:400–4.

156 Schiere S, Proost JH, Schuringa M, Wierda JMKH. Pharmacokinetics and pharmacokinetic-dynamic relationship between rapacuronium (ORG 9487), and its 3-desacetyl metabolite (ORG 9488). *Anesth Analg* 1999;**88**:640–7.

157 Boyd AH, Eastwood NB, Parker CJR, Hunter JM. Comparison of the pharmacodynamics and pharmacokinetics of an infusion of *cis*-atracurium (51W89) or atracurium in critically ill patients undergoing mechanical ventilation in an intensive therapy unit. *Br J Anaesth* 1996;**76**:382–8.

158 Prielipp RC, Coursin DB, Scuderi PE *et al.* Comparison of the infusion requirements

and recovery profiles of vecuronium and cisatracurium (51W89) in intensive care unit patients. *Anesth Analg* 1995;81:3–12.

159 Segredo V, Matthay MA, Sharma ML, Gruenke LD, Caldwell JE, Miller RD. Prolonged neuromuscular blockade after long-term administration of vecuronium in two critically ill patients. *Anesthesiology* 1990;72:566–70.

160 Segredo V, Caldwell JE, Wright PM, Sharma ML, Gruenke LD, Miller RD. Do the pharmacokinetics of vecuronium change during prolonged administration in critically ill patients? *Br J Anaesth* 1998; 80:707–9.

161 Partridge BL, Abrams JH, Bazemore C, Rubin R. Prolonged neuromuscular blockade after long-term infusion of vecuronium bromide in the intensive care unit. *Crit Care Med* 1990;18:1177–9.

162 Gooch JL, Suchyta MR, Balbierz JM, Petajan JH, Clemmer TP. Prolonged paralysis after treatment with neuromuscular junction blocking agents. *Crit Care Med* 1991;19:1125–31.

163 Welling PG, Craig WA, Amidon GL, Kunin CM. Pharmacokinetics of cefazolin in normal ands uremic subjects. *Clin Pharmacol Ther* 1974;15:344–53.

164 Welling PG, Shaw WTR, Uman SJ, Tse FCS, Craig WG. Phamacokinetics of minocycline in renal failure. *Antimicrob Agents Chemother* 1975;8:532–7.

165 Sladen RN, Endo E, Harrison T. Two hour versus twenty-two hour creatinine clearance in critically ill patients. *Anesthesiology* 1987;67:1013–16.

166 Hofmann W, Kroh H, Lennartz H. Infection-induced changes in the pharmacokinetics of cefotaxime. Dose calculation in multiple organ failure and relevance of score systems. *Klin Wochenschr* 1991; 69, suppl 26:32–5.

167 van Dalen R, Vree TB, Baars AM, Termond E. Dose adjustment of ceftazidine in patients with impaired renal function. *Eur J Clin Pharmacol* 1986;30:597–605.

168 Schumach GE. Pharmacokinetic analysis of gentamicin dosage regimes for renal impairment. *J Clin Pharmacol* 1975;15:656–65.

169 Zaske DE, Cipolle RJ, Strate RJ. Gentamicin dosage requirements: wide interpatient variation in 242 surgery patients with normal renal function. *Surgery* 1980;87:164–9.

170 Sawchuk RJ, Zaske DE, Cipolle RJ. Kinetic model for gentamicin dosing with the use of individual patient parameters. *Clin Pharmacol Ther* 1977;21:362–5.

171 Hickling K, Begg E, Moore ML. A prospective randomised trial comparing individualised pharmacokinetic dosage prediction for aminoglycosides with prediction based on estimated creatinine clearance in critically ill patients. *Intens Care Med* 1989;15:233–7.

172 Mitchell PR, Wilson J, Dodek P, Russell JA. Volume of distribution in patients with gram negative sepsis in the ICU. *Anesthesiology* 1987;67:A126 (abstract).

173 Watling SM, Kisor DF. Population pharmacokinetics: development of a medical intensive care unit-specific gentamicin dosing nomogram. *Ann Pharmacother* 1993;27:151–4.

174 Boldt J, Salomon P, Krumholz W, Hempelmann G. Effect of continuous mechanical hemofiltration on the pharmacokinetics of antibiotics exemplified by mezlocillin. *Anasth Intensivther Notfallmed* 1988;23:91–4.

175 Schetz M, Ferdinande P, Van den Berghe G, Verwaest CM, Lauwers P. Pharmacokinetics of continuous renal replacement therapy. *Intens Care Med* 1995;21:612–20.

176 Gwilt PR, Perrier D. Plasma protein binding and distribution characteristics of drugs as indices of their hemodialyzability. *Clin Pharmacol Ther* 1978;24:154–61.

177 Kulka PJ, Tryba M. Inotropic support of the critically ill patient: a review of the agents. *Drugs* 1993;45:654–67.

178 Le Corre P, Malledant Y, Tanguy M, Le Verge R. Steady-state pharmacokinetics of dopamine in adult patients. *Crit Care Med* 1993;21:1652–7.

179 Doherty J, Flanigan WJ, Perkins WH, Ackerman GL. Studies with tritiated digoxin in anephric human subjects. *Circulation* 1967;35:298–303.

180 Oetgen WJ, Sobol SM, Tri TB, Heydom WH, Rakita L. Amiodarone–digoxin interactions: clinical and experimental observations. *Chest* 1984;86:75–9.

181 Graves SW, Brown B, Valdes R. An endogenous digoxin like substance in patients with renal impairment. *Arch Intern Med* 1983;99:604–8.

5: Hepatic failure

FELICITY HAWKER

The liver is the principal site of drug metabolism. It is therefore not surprising that hepatic failure has significant effects on the pharmacokinetics of therapeutic drugs. Other manifestations of hepatic failure (for example, hypoalbuminaemia) may have additional or opposite effects on drug disposition and drug effects.

The term "hepatic failure" typically is used to describe the fulminant liver failure associated with the various causes of acute hepatic necrosis and also the end stage of a number of chronic liver diseases of which cirrhosis is one of the most common. For the purposes of this chapter, cholestasis, the systemic inflammatory response syndrome (SIRS), and its hepatic manifestation – "ICU jaundice" – and ischaemic hepatitis will also be discussed. These latter conditions occur in the critically ill but cannot be classified as hepatic failure.

The effects of liver disease on drug handling are variable and depend to an extent upon the type of liver disease.[1] Most of the published work concerns patients with cirrhosis, and for this reason this chapter examines this group in the most detail. However, the most important factor is disease severity. In broad terms, there is a relationship between the degree of derangement of drug handling and degree of liver impairment.[2] Unfortunately there are no sensitive and specific criteria that correlate with the severity of liver function impairment, and adjustment of drug dosage in patients with liver failure depends on an understanding of the many factors discussed below.

Drug absorption

Altered absorption of drugs from the gastrointestinal tract is not thought to be a major factor affecting drug disposition in patients with hepatic failure, although the subject has not been well studied. Certainly, patients with cirrhosis frequently complain of gastrointestinal symptoms, and also have an increased incidence of problems such as peptic ulcer and gastritis. This group has been shown to have delayed gastric emptying (approximately double that in healthy controls).[3] Abnormal levels of gastrointestinal peptides such as glucagon, cholecystokinin or motilin, rather than autonomic dysfunction, are the likely cause. Altered gut motility has also been implicated as the cause of slower than normal absorption of frusemide in patients with cirrhosis,[4] although the extent of absorption appears to be normal. There is also evidence that absorption of the β-blocker bisoprolol is impaired in advanced chronic liver disease,[5] an effect that compensates to an extent for the impairment of its metabolism.

In cholestatic liver disease, reduced bile acids in the intestine may impair drug absorption.

Drug distribution

Volume of distribution

Patients with advanced chronic liver disease have an increased total body water because of oedema and ascites. Drugs that are distributed in total body water, such as the non-depolarising muscle relaxants, will be distributed in a larger volume, and peak levels with normal doses are likely to be subtherapeutic. This is the probable explanation of the resistance to these agents noted in advanced liver disease.[6,7] Similar problems may complicate the use of aminoglycoside antibiotics. Difficulty in obtaining therapeutic peak levels, in addition to enhanced nephrotoxicity in chronic liver disease,[8,9] make aminoglycosides very difficult to use and they are best avoided. Many other drugs, for example propranolol, have an increased volume of distribution in patients with ascites.[10]

Protein binding

Liver disease can influence the binding of drugs in plasma in a number of ways. These include the decrease in plasma albumin concentration seen in chronic hepatic failure, the presence of altered or defective plasma proteins, and displacement of drugs from binding sites by a variety of endogenous and exogenous compounds, such as bilirubin.

In theory, whatever the reason, reduced binding to plasma proteins increases the availability of the total drug concentration in the blood for uptake into tissues and may therefore result in an increased effect. It will also increase the amount of drug presented to the liver and kidneys for elimination. In general, the effect of liver disease on drug binding is most marked in patients with advanced liver disease, and when the drug in question is highly protein bound. Overall, these effects are minor in comparison with changes that result from altered drug elimination in patients with liver disease. As discussed in Chapter 2, humans with an hereditary inability to synthesise albumin can maintain relatively good health.

Drug elimination

Metabolism

Drug metabolism by the liver is dependent upon both liver blood flow and the intrinsic activity of the hepatic enzymes involved. As discussed in Chapter 2, drugs that are avidly metabolised by the liver (high extraction

Table 5.1   Classification by hepatic extraction of some commonly used drugs.

	Drug	Estimated hepatic extraction (%)	$t_{1/2}$ health (h)	$t_{1/2}$ liver disease (h)	Fraction cleared by liver
Blood flow limited or high-extraction drugs	Lignocaine	72	1·5	1·6	96
	Verapamil	85	3·7	14	100
	Propranolol	80	2·9	7·7	100
	Morphine	77	2·5	2·2	90
	Amitriptyline	65	16	38	98
	Chlormethiazole	76	6·6	8·7	95
Enzyme limited or low-extraction drugs	Diazepam	2	47	105	100
	Phenobarbitone	1	99	?	76
	Phenytoin	1–3	14–50	13	95
	Warfarin	1	25	23	100
	Antipyrine	3	10	27	95
	Caffeine	4	5·2	6·1	80
	Chloramphenicol	11	4·6	11	90
Flow and enzyme sensitive or intermediate-extraction drugs	Aspirin	50	0·3	?	99
	Paracetamol	31	2·0	3·1	96
	Pethidine	55	5·2	11	98
	Fentanyl	53	4·4	5·1	94
	Nifedipine	50	1·9	7	100
	Haloperidol	55	20	?	100

Modified from Bircher and Sharifi.[11]

ratio) are most affected by changes in liver blood flow, and their metabolism is reduced when blood flow is reduced. Drugs with a low extraction ratio are little influenced by changes in blood flow but instead are dependent upon the metabolic capacity of the relevant enzyme. Common examples of drugs with high, low and intermediate extraction ratios are shown in Table 5.1.

Liver blood flow

There are characteristic changes in liver blood flow in chronic liver disease. These include reduced overall flow, and there may also be redistribution of flow within the lobule because of scarring due to cirrhosis and/or portal systemic shunting (up to 60% of portal blood flow can pass to the systemic circulation through these shunts)[12]. Cirrhotic diseases have the greatest effect on liver blood flow and drugs with high extraction ratios are most affected. Changes are less marked in other types of hepatic failure.

These characteristic changes result in high peak drug concentrations when high-extraction drugs are given orally. Because of the possibility of overdosage, these drugs have been called "high-risk" agents. The dose rather than the frequency should be reduced if these drugs are prescribed for patients with liver disease. The pharmacokinetic profile of high-extraction drugs is less abnormal in patients with liver disease when they are given parenterally, although reduced hepatic uptake and intrahepatic shunting may still lead to elevated blood levels.[13] Drugs may alter their own pharmacokinetics if they alter liver blood flow. For example, the clearance of the active D-isomer of propranolol is lower than that of the inactive isomer because of its negative effect on cardiac output.[14] A similar phenomenon is seen with verapamil. On the other hand, glucagon and isoprenaline increase the clearance of lignocaine and propranolol because they increase liver blood flow.[15]

Activity of microsomal enzymes in liver disease

This depends to an extent on the nature of the liver disease, its severity and the drug in question. A number of model drugs have been used to assess microsomal enzyme function. These include antipyrine, aminopyrine, caffeine, galactose, indocyanine green, lignocaine, and erythromycin. Enzyme activity can also be measured directly in liver tissue.

Enzyme function is most influenced by hepatocellular diseases. These conditions will therefore mostly affect those drugs with low extraction ratios for which hepatic clearance is essentially dependent upon the metabolic capacity of the liver. The pharmacokinetic profiles of low-extraction drugs tend to show increased half-life rather than high peak blood levels in patients with liver disease. Theoretically, the dosage interval should be increased, rather than the dose decreased. However, several sedatives are included in this group and they may have heightened effects in patients with liver disease because of increased end-organ sensitivity[15] and the dose should be reduced for this reason.

When the extraction of a drug is intermediate, the clearance from the blood may be sensitive to changes in both liver blood flow and enzyme activity.

Altered drug metabolism in liver failure is also dependent to an extent on the type of liver disease or failure present.

Chronic liver disease

The activity of drug-metabolising enzymes is decreased in patients with chronic liver disease, and in general, the reduction parallels the severity of the disease.[16] The type of liver disease present also has some effect on the degree of impairment of drug metabolism. This can be severe with cirrhosis but patients with chronic active hepatitis and primary biliary cirrhosis have only mild to moderate impairment of hepatic oxidative drug metabolism. In addition, the clearance of different drugs may vary in the same patient because all metabolic pathways are not affected equally by liver disease. Oxidation of drugs is carried out principally by the cytochromes P450 (CYP) that are situated predominantly in zone 3 (centrilobular area) of the hepatic lobule. By contrast, enzymes responsible for conjugation (such as the glucuronyl transferases) are plentiful in zone 1 (periportal area). Enzymes situated in zone 3, an area more prone to hypoxia, appear to be more affected in liver disease than those in zone 1, and there is some evidence that glucuronidation is reasonably well preserved in patients with cirrhosis when compared with oxidation.[17] The elimination of drugs that are primarily metabolised by conjugation with glucuronic acid (morphine, lorazepam, oxazepam) may consequently be unaltered, even in patients who have impaired oxidative metabolism.[18] Data on other conjugation pathways such as sulphation and acetylation are limited and somewhat conflicting.[2] Even more specifically, different cytochromes P450 may be affected to different degrees in the same patient.[19] In a study of a group of patients with mild or moderate liver disease, there was a 79% decrease in plasma clearance of a drug metabolised by CYP 2C19 (S-mephenytoin), but no effect on a drug metabolised by CYP 2D6 (debrisoquine). Since different groups of drugs are oxidised by different cytochromes, knowledge of the enzyme involved in the metabolism of a specific drug may become important for recommended dose modifications in hepatic failure. However, further studies of individual drug-metabolising enzymes in the presence of disease are required.

Other factors such as malnutrition, common in chronic hepatic failure, may contribute to the impairment of drug metabolism.[20]

Increases in the volume of distribution of drugs distributed in total body water because of ascites and oedema, decreased plasma protein binding because of hypoalbuminaemia, changes in liver blood flow, and portal systemic shunting also alter the effects of drugs in patients with chronic liver disease. As discussed later, drugs excreted by the kidneys will also have reduced clearance, whether or not overt renal failure is present.

Acute liver failure

In acute liver failure, metabolic ability of liver is severely impaired due to reduction of the mass of functionally active liver cells because of extensive liver cell necrosis. The degree of functional impairment is related to the severity of the liver injury. For example, antipyrine clearance is subnormal in patients with acute liver failure and patients with the most severe reductions have the highest mortality rates.[21] Studies of the metabolism of individual drugs show there is reduced metabolism of pethidine, hexobarbitone and chlordiazepoxide in acute hepatitis,[22] whereas the clearance of tolbutamide, warfarin, and phenytoin has been shown to be normal.[23] It is most likely these inconsistencies reflect different degrees of liver failure in different studies, rather than differential effects of hepatocyte necrosis on oxidative enzyme systems. It is reasonable to assume that all drugs metabolised by the liver will have reduced clearance in patients with acute liver failure. In this circumstance, the probability of enhanced and prolonged drug effects should be anticipated, and drugs should only be given if they are thought to be absolutely necessary.

Obstructive jaundice and cholestatic liver disease

Although drug metabolism in patients with obstructive jaundice is generally less impaired than with acute and chronic liver failure, animal studies show there can be a 50% reduction in hepatic cytochrome P450 content after bile duct ligation.[24] This is believed to be caused by increased intrahepatic bile acid concentrations associated with obstructive jaundice. In keeping with these findings, studies of patients with cholestasis show they have reduced clearance of a number of drugs[25] and reduced hepatic cytochrome P450 content.[26] Moreover, cholestasis is associated with a different pattern of hepatic P450 expression. 1A is reduced, 2E1 and 3A are differentially affected, whereas 2C is unaltered except in pronounced cases of cholestasis.

In addition to these effects on drug metabolism, both intra- and extra-hepatic cholestasis prolong the effects of drugs for which biliary excretion is the major elimination route. On the other hand, the absence of bile salts in the bowel can result in reduced absorption of some drugs when given orally and consequently reduced effects. Plasma protein binding of some drugs may be reduced due to competition with bile salts.

Overall, drug disposition, the choice of drug, and drug dosage are affected by the same considerations as have been outlined above, although the effects of obstructive jaundice and other cholestatic conditions are less pronounced.

"ICU jaundice"[27]/systemic inflammatory response syndrome (SIRS)

Drug metabolism in "ICU jaundice" has not been widely studied. Microsomal enzyme activity has been shown to be reduced in experimental models of trauma,[28] endotoxin administration,[29] and severe burns.[30] These findings are probably the result of inhibition of cytochrome P450 enzymes by conditions such as hypoxia[31] and endogenous substances, such as interferon,[32] interleukin-1,[33] interleukin-6,[34] and other cytokines. Phase II enzymes may also be affected. Impaired drug handling has also been found in patients with trauma[35] and burns[36] and normal individuals injected with endotoxin.[37] It is not clear whether these findings reflect only a reduced metabolic capacity of the liver, or additional changes in hepatic blood flow, protein binding, and drug excretion that can occur in critical illness. Although impaired drug handling is clearly present in these jaundiced critically ill patients, data are lacking and no recommendations regarding drug dosage can be made at present.

Ischaemic hepatitis

Animal studies suggest that oxidative metabolism of drugs may be reduced in experimental haemorrhagic shock.[38] Although there are no studies of patients with ischaemic hepatitis, it is likely the capacity for hepatic drug metabolism is reduced in this group. More importantly, patients with ischaemic hepatitis have reduced liver blood flow by definition. Drugs with high hepatic extraction that are metabolised chiefly in the liver will therefore have enhanced effects when given orally. This group of drugs includes some β-blockers, calcium channel antagonists and antiarrhythmic drugs that are commonly prescribed for patients with heart disease. Because these drugs are cardiac depressants, reductions in their clearance because of decreased liver blood flow will further reduce liver blood flow, further reduce their clearance, and magnify their adverse effects on the circulation. This mechanism has been proposed as a reason for the high mortality of patients with ischaemic hepatitis treated with these drugs.[39]

Miscellaneous liver diseases

The metabolism of antipyrine is normal in patients with extensive metastatic liver involvement,[40] suggesting that modification of drug doses is not necessary in this group. Patients with other liver diseases have not been widely studied but it is unlikely that drug disposition would be significantly altered unless hepatic failure or cirrhosis is present.

Extrahepatic metabolism

Although the liver plays the major role in drug metabolism, it should be remembered that drug-metabolising enzymes are present at other sites (see Chapter 2) and can contribute to drug elimination, depending upon the circumstances.[41] Thus extrahepatic metabolism may be responsible for the clearance of some drugs even when there is severe hepatic failure or when the patient is anhepatic.

Excretion

Biliary excretion It is clear that drugs eliminated in the bile (conjugates with glucuronic acid, organic cations, and some steroids) will accumulate when there is extrahepatic biliary obstruction and intrahepatic cholestasis. Although data are scanty, it seems that there is also reduced biliary clearance of a number of drugs in patients with cirrhosis.

Renal excretion Renal impairment (characteristically the hepatorenal syndrome) is a common accompaniment of end-stage liver disease and it is not surprising that renal drug clearance will be impaired in this setting. However, even moderate degrees of hepatic impairment can be associated with a decrease in renal clearance of drugs or active drug metabolites normally excreted by the kidney. Therefore drugs cleared renally as well as those cleared hepatically may need dosage modification in patients with liver failure. Assessments of renal function based on creatinine, particularly serum creatinine concentration, may greatly overestimate renal drug clearance in patients with hepatic failure.[2]

Drug interactions in liver disease

Some drugs may effect the metabolism of other drugs either by induction or inhibition of drug-metabolising enzymes. Phenobarbitone, phenytoin, rifampicin, spironolactone, and some other drugs induce the synthesis of drug-metabolising enzymes and result in increased clearance of other drugs given at the same time. Administration of these drugs may offset, to an extent, reductions in cytochrome P450 enzyme activity due to liver disease, although the liver's reserve capacity in advanced liver disease is probably too limited for these drugs to exert any significant effect. On the other hand, the effects of drugs such as cimetidine that inhibit the oxidative metabolism of many drugs, such as theophylline[42] may further limit the metabolic capacity of the failing liver.

Pharmacodynamics in liver disease

Changes in the response to a given concentration of drug in plasma can arise from either altered drug access to the site of action (for example, decreased plasma protein binding, altered blood–brain barrier permeability) or altered receptor sensitivity.

Important pharmacodynamic changes in liver failure include:

- increased sensitivity to sedatives and strong analgesics
- decreased sensitivity to adrenergic agents.

Increased sensitivity to sedatives and strong analgesics

Patients with hepatic failure are exquisitely sensitive to sedative agents[43] and treatment with such drugs is a recognised precipitant of hepatic encephalopathy. There is experimental evidence of increased permeability of the blood–brain barrier in hepatic failure[44] that may increase access of sedative agents into the brain. As discussed earlier, decreased protein binding could contribute to this effect. However, the most important cause of the increased sensitivity to sedatives and analgesics in patients with liver failure is likely to be a change in the density and affinity of cerebral receptors for these agents. For example, there is evidence for increased binding at the central benzodiazepine receptor in patients with hepatic encephalopathy.[45] This is greatest in the thalamus, cerebelium, and pons. It is a likely cause for the increased sensitivity of patients with hepatic failure to the sedative effects of benzodiazepine drugs.

Decreased sensitivity to adrenergic agents

Plasma catecholamine levels are increased in both acute and chronic liver failure.[46,47] This chronic sympathetic stimulation is probably the cause of the down-regulation of adrenergic receptors observed in cirrhosis and other forms of decompensated liver disease, which leads to inotrope resistance. For example, it has been known for some time that patients with chronic liver disease have impaired vascular responsiveness to noradrenaline.[48] More recently, Ramond et al.[49] found that the dose of isoprenaline required to induce an increase in heart rate of 25 beats/min in cirrhotics was almost four times that required for controls. This mechanism is also responsible for the decreased sensitivity observed to adrenergic antagonists (for example, the non-selective β-blocker metipranolol)[50]. The mechanism of the diuretic resistance[51] that is seen in patients with cirrhosis is not so clear.

96

Examples of altered pharmacology in liver disease

Benzodiazepines

Midazolam is the benzodiazepine that has been studied most extensively in patients with liver disease. It is metabolised by CYP 3A to hydroxy and dihydroxy metabolites. Although different liver diseases may affect the amount of the enzyme and therefore the rate of metabolism of midazolam to different degrees,[1] overall there is reduced clearance in the presence of liver disease with a prolongation of the elimination half-life. Other benzodiazepines that are metabolised by oxidation are affected similarly. However, benzodiazepines that are metabolised by conjugation with glucuronic acid (oxazepam, temazepam, lorazepam) have relatively normal pharmacokinetics in liver disease and are preferred agents in this setting. Nevertheless even these safer drugs should be given at a reduced dose. This is because of the heightened cerebral response to these drugs in liver disease[43,52] due to alteration of the receptor–concentration relationship so that a given effect is elicited by smaller concentrations of the drug.

β-Adrenergic blockers

The pharmacology of propranolol (and to a lesser extent other β-blockers) has been studied widely in patients with liver disease because of its use in the treatment of portal hypertension and to reduce the risk of bleeding from oesophageal varices. Many factors interact to determine the fate of ingested propranolol in liver disease. On the one hand, mean steady-state unbound propranolol concentration was found to be increased three-fold in a group of patients with well-compensated cirrhosis compared with healthy controls.[53] This is most likely due to a combination of portosystemic vascular shunts allowing more of the absorbed drug to reach the systemic circulation, reduced metabolism, and perhaps reduced protein binding. It is possible that reduced absorption may slightly counterbalance these effects.[5] Similar pharmacokinetic findings have been reported for other β-blockers.[54,55] On the other hand, there seems to be a reduction in receptor sensitivity so that higher steady-state drug concentration is required to achieve the same effect.[50]

Despite these conflicting factors, the net result is that the effects of the drug will be increased. The initial dose should be reduced and then increased stepwise until a physiologically appropriate end point is reached, for example, reduction of heart rate by 25%.

β-Lactam antibiotics

Penicillins are largely renally excreted and therefore liver disease has little effect on their pharmacokinetics. However, for the acylureidopenicillins (for example, piperacillin), 50% of the systemic clearance is non-renal and there is an increased elimination half-life in patients with liver disease.[56] It is therefore appropriate to reduce the dose (by about half) or increase the dosage interval when using acylureidopenicillins in patients with marked hepatic impairment. The third-generation cephalosporins (cefotaxime, ceftriaxone) also have significant non-renal clearance under normal circumstances, but in the presence of liver disease there is a compensatory increase in renal clearance such that no dosage modification is necessary unless there is additional impairment of renal function.

Conclusion

There is no single reliable method for prediction of optimal drug doses in patients with liver disease and "safe" drug use requires consideration of the many factors discussed in this chapter. However, some generalisations can be made:

- Drugs with high hepatic extraction that are metabolised chiefly by the liver will have enhanced effects if given orally at normal doses.
- Drugs with low hepatic extraction that are metabolised chiefly by the liver will accumulate if given at normal dosage intervals.
- Drugs distributed in total body water may need higher loading doses in the presence of ascites and oedema.
- There are enhanced pharmacological responses to benzodiazepines and probably to barbiturates and narcotic analgesics, that are independent of changes in pharmacokinetics.
- Angiotensin converting enzyme inhibitors,[57] non-steroidal anti-inflammatory drugs,[58] and aminoglycoside antibiotics[8,9] have increased nephrotoxicity in patients with liver disease and can cause renal failure.
- When prodrugs require conversion to the active molety by metabolism in the liver [angioterisin converting enzyme (ACE) inhibitors and methylprednisolone hemisuccinate], the rate of formation of active drug may be decreased, resulting in a lesser effect.[2]

Individual drugs that are probably safe, should have the dose reduced or the dosage interval increased, or be avoided altogether are shown in Table 5.2. Overall, drugs should be carefully selected, doses should err on the side of caution, plasma levels should be monitored and the possibility of drug toxicity should be anticipated.[59]

Table 5.2 Examples of drugs that are probably safe, require dose reduction, or should be avoided in patients with hepatic failure.

Drug class	Probably safe	Reduce dose or dosage interval	Avoid
Analgesics	Paracetamol	Narcotic analgesics	Aspirin NSAIDs
Sedatives	Oxazepam Lorazepam Temazepam	Diazepam Midazolam	Zopiclone
Antihypertensives and other cardiovascular	Clonidine Digoxin	Propranolol Metoprolol Verapamil Nifedipine Diltiazem Flecainide Lignocaine Mexilitine Quinidine	ACE inhibitors
Anticonvulsants	Phenobarbitone	Phenytoin Valproic acid	
Antiulcer	Omeprazole Ranitidine	Famotidine	Cimetidine
Antiemetic		Metoclopramide Ondansetron	
Antibiotics	Penicillins Cephalosporins Fluconazole	Ureidopenicillins Fluoroquinolones Vancomycin Erythromycin Metronidazole	Aminoglycosides

Adapted from Westphal and Brogard[60]
ACE, angiotensin converting enzyme; NSAID, non-steroidal anti-inflammatory drug

1 Park GR, Miller E. What changes drug metabolism in critically ill patients-III? Effect of pre-existing disease on the metabolism of midazolam. *Anaesthesia* 1996;51:431–4.
2 Morgan DJ, McLean AJ. Clinical pharmacokinetic and pharmacodynamic considerations in patients with liver disease. *Clin Pharmacokinet* 1995;29:370–91.
3 Isobe H, Sakai H, Satoh M, Sakamoto S, Nawata H. Delayed gastric emptying in patients with liver cirrhosis. *Dig Dis Sci* 1994;39:983–7.
4 Fredrick MJ, Pound DC, Hall SD, Brater DC. Furosemide absorption in patients with cirrhosis. *Clin Pharmacol Ther* 1991;49:241–7.
5 Hayes PC, Jenkins D, Vavianos P *et al.* Single dose pharmacokinetics of bisoprolol in liver disease. *Eur Heart J* 1987;8 (suppl M):23–9.
6 Dundee JW, Gray TC. Resistance to *d*-tubocurarine in presence of liver damage. *Lancet* 1953;ii:16–17.
7 Ward ME, Adu-Gyanfi Y, Strunin L. Althesin and pancuronium in chronic liver disease. *Br J Anaesth* 1975;47:1199–204.
8 Cabrera J, Arroyo V, Bailesta A *et al.* Aminoglycoside nephrotoxicity in cirrhosis. Value of urinary β2-microglobulin to discriminate functional renal failure from tubular damage. *Gastroenterology* 1982;82:97–105.
9 Moore RD, Smith CR, Lipsky JJ, Mellits ED, Lietman PS. Risk factors for nephrotoxicity in patients treated with aminoglycosides. *Ann Intern Med* 1984;100:352–7.

10 Branch RA, James J, Read AE. A study of factors influencing drug disposition in chronic liver disease using the model drug (+)-propranolol. *Br J Clin Pharmacol* 1976;3:243–9.

11 Bircher J, Sharifi S. Drug dosage in patients with liver disease. In: McIntyre N, Benhamou J-P, Bircher J, Rizzetto M, Rodes J, eds. *Oxford textbook of clinical hepatology.* Oxford: Oxford University Press, 1991 : 1388–400.

12 Syrota A, Paraf A, Gaudebout C, Desgreez A. Significance of intra- and extra-hepatic portasystemic shunting in survival of cirrhotic patients. *Dig Dis Sci* 1981;26:878–85.

13 Pessayre D, Lebrec D, Descatoire V, Peignoux P, Benhamou J-P. Mechanism for reducing blood clearance in patients with cirrhosis. *Gastroenterology* 1978;74:566–71.

14 Wilkinson GR, Shand DG. A physiologic approach to hepatic drug clearance. *Clin Pharmacol Ther* 1975;18:370–90.

15 Hayes PC. Liver disease and drug disposition. *Br J Anaesth* 1992;68:459–61.

16 Villeneuve JP, Infante-Rivard C, Ampelas M, Pomier-Layrargues G, Huet PM, Marieau D. Prognostic value of the aminopyrine breath test in cirrhotic patients *Hepatology* 1986;6:928–31.

17 Hoyumpa AM, Shenker S. Is glucuronidation truly preserved in patients with liver disease? *Hepatology* 1991;13:786–95.

18 Shull HJ, Wilkinson GR, Johnson R, Schenker S. Normal disposition of oxazepam in acute viral hepatitis and cirrhosis. *Ann Intern Med* 1976;84:420–5.

19 Adedoyin A, Arns PA, Richards WO, Wilkinson GR, Branch RA. Selective effect of liver disease on the activities of specific metabolizing enzymes: investigation of cytochromes P450 2C19 and 2D6. *Clin Pharmacol Ther* 1998;64:8–17.

20 Pantuck EJ, Pantuck C, Weissman C, Gil KM, Askanazi J. Stimulation of oxidative drug metabolism by parenteral refeeding of nutritionally depleted patients. *Gastroenterology* 1985;89:241–5.

21 Tygstrup N, Ranek L. Assessment of prognosis in fulminant hepatic failure. *Semin Liver Dis* 1986;6:129–37.

22 McHorse TS, Wilkinson GR, Johnson RF, Schenker S. Effect of acute viral hepatitis in man on the disposition and elimination of meperidine. *Gastroenterology* 1975;68:775–80.

23 Blaschke TF, Meffin PJ, Melmon KL, Rowland M. Influence of acute viral hepatitis on phenytoin kinetics and protein binding. *Clin Pharmacol Ther* 1975;17:685–91.

24 Mackinnon AM, Simon FR. Reduced synthesis of hepatic microsomal cytochrome P450 in the bile duct ligated rat. *Biochem Biophys Res Commun* 1974;56:437–43.

25 Kato R. Drug metabolism under pathological and abnormal physical states in animals and man. *Xenobiotica* 1977;7:25–92.

26 Kawata S, Imai Y, Inada M *et al.* Selective reduction of hepatic cytochrome P450 content in patients with intrahepatic cholestasis: a mechanism for impairment of microsomal drug oxidation. *Gastroenterology* 1987;92:299–303.

27 Hawker F. Liver dysfunction in critical illness. *Anaesth Intens Care* 1991;19:165–81.

28 Rauckman E, Rosen G, Post S, Gillogly S. Effect of model traumatic injury on hepatic drug metabolising enzymes. *J Trauma* 1980;20:884–6.

29 Sowane B, Yaffe S. Effects of endotoxin upon rat hepatic microsomal drug metabolism *in vivo* and *in vitro. Xenobiotica* 1982;12:303–13.

30 Frunicillo R, DiGregorio G. The effect of thermal injury on drug metabolism in the rat. *J Trauma* 1983;23:523–9.

31 Park GR, Pichard L, Tinel M *et al.* What changes drug metabolism in critically ill patients? Two preliminary studies in isolated human hepatocytes. *Anaesthesia* 1994;49:188–9.

32 Singh G, Renton KW. Interferon-mediated depression of cytochrome P450-dependent drug biotransformation. *Mol Pharmacol* 1981;20:681–4.

33 Ghezzi P, Saccardo B, Villa P, Rossi V, Bianchi M, Dinarello C. Role of interleukin-1 in the depression of liver drug metabolism by endotoxin. *Infect Immun* 1986;54:837–40.

34 Gurley BJ, Barone GW, Yamashita K, Polston S, Estes M, Harden A. Extrahepatic ischemia-reperfusion injury reduces hepatic oxidative drug metabolism as determined by serial antipyrine clearance. *Pharmacol Res* 1997;14:67–72.

35 Slaughter R, Hassett J. Hepatic drug clearance following traumatic injury. *Drug Intell Clin Pharmacol* 1985;19:799–806.

36 Ciaccio E, Frunicillo R. Urinary excretion of D-glucaric acid by severely burned patients. *Clin Pharmacol Ther* 1979;25:340–4.

37 Shedlofsky SI, Israel BC, Tosheva R, Blouin RA. Endotoxin depresses hepatic cytochrome P450 drug metabolism in women. *Br J Clin Pharmacol* 1997;43:627–32.

38 DiPiro JT, Hooker KD, Sherman JC, Gaines M, Wynne JJ. Effect of experimental hemorrhagic shock on hepatic drug elimination. *Crit Care Med* 1992;20:810–15.

100

39 Potter JM, Hickman PE. Cardiodepressant drugs and the high mortality rate associated with ischaemic hepatitis. *Crit Care Med* 1992;**20**:474–8.

40 Robertz-Vaupel GM, Lindecken KD, Edeki T, Funke C, Belwon S, Dengler HJ. Disposition of antipyrine in patients with extensive metastatic liver disease. *Eur J Clin Pharmacol* 1992;**42**:465–9.

41 Krishna DR, Klotz U. Extrahepatic metabolism of drugs in humans. *Clin Pharmacokinet* 1994;**26**:144–60.

42 Nelson DC, Avant GR, Speeg KV Jr, Hoyumpa AM Jr, Schenker S. The effect of cimetidine on hepatic drug elimination in cirrhosis. *Hepatology* 1985;**5**:305–9.

43 Branch RA, Morgan MH, James J, Reid AE. Intravenous administration of diazepam in patients with chronic liver disease. *Gut* 1976;**17**:975–83.

44 Zaki AE, Ede RJ, Davis M, Williams R. Experimental studies of blood–brain barrier permeability in acute hepatic failure. *Hepatology* 1984;**4**:359–63.

45 Macdonald GA, Frey KA, Agranoff BW *et al*. Cerebral benzodiazepine receptor binding *in vivo* in patients with recurrent hepatic encephalopathy. *Hepatology* 1997;**26**:277–82.

46 Ring Larsen H, Hesse B, Henriksen JH, Christensen NJ. Sympathetic nervous activity and renal and systemic haemodynamics in cirrhosis: plasma norepinephrine concentration, hepatic extraction and renal disease. *Hepatology* 1982;**2**:304–10.

47 Bihari DJ, Gimson AES, Williams R. Disturbances in cardiovascular and pulmonary function in fulminant hepatic failure. In: Williams R, ed. *Clinics in critical care medicine*: liver failure. London: Churchill Livingstone, 1986;47–71.

48 Lunzer M, Manghani K, Newman S, Sherlock S, Bernard A, Ginsberg J. Impaired cardiovascular responsiveness in liver disease. *Lancet* 1975;**ii**:382–5.

49 Ramond MJ, Comoy E, Lebrec D. Alterations in isoprenaline sensitivity of patients with cirrhosis: evidence of abnormality of the sympathetic nervous activity. *Br J Clin Pharmacol* 1986;**21**:191–6.

50 Janku I, Perlik F, Tkaczykova M, Brodanova M. Disposition effects and concentration effect relationship of metipranolol in patients with cirrhosis and healthy subjects. *Eur J Clin Pharmacol* 1992;**42**:337–40.

51 Schwartz S, Brater DC, Pound D, Green PK, Kramer WG, Rudy D. Bioavailability, pharmacokinetcs, and pharmacodynamics of torsemide in patients with cirrhosis. *Clin Pharmacol Ther* 1993;**54**:90–7.

52 Bakti G, Fisch HU, Kariaganis G, Minder C, Bircher J. Mechanism of the excessive sedative response of cirrhotics to benzodiazepines: model experiments with triazolam. *Hepatology* 1987;**7**:629–38.

53 Wood AJ, Kornhauser DM, Wilkinson GR, Shand DG, Branch RA. The influence of cirrhosis on steady state blood concentrations of unbound propranolol after oral administration. *Clin Pharmacokinet* 1978;**3**:478–87.

54 Regardh CG, Jordo L, Ervik M, Lundborg P, Olsson R, Ronn O. Pharmacokinetics of metoprolol in patients with hepatic cirrhosis. *Clin Pharmacokinet* 1981;**6**:375–88.

55 Cales P, Caillau H, Crambes O *et al*. Hemodynamic and pharmacokinetic study of tertolol in patients with alcoholic cirrhosis and portal hypertension. *J Hepatol* 1993;**19**:43–50.

56 Bunke CM, Aronoff BR, Brier ME, Sloan RS, Luft FC. Mezlocillin kinetics in hepatic insufficiency. *Clin Pharmacol Ther* 1983;**33**:73–6.

57 Daskalopoulos G, Pinzani M, Murray N, Hirschberb R, Zipser RD. Effects of captopril on renal function in patients with cirrhosis and ascites. *J Hepatol* 1987;**4**:330–6.

58 Laffi G, Daskalopoulos G, Kronberg I, Hsueh W, Gentilini P, Zipser RD. Effects of sulindac and ibuprofen in patients with cirrhosis and ascites: an explanation for the renal sparing effect of sulindac. *Gastroenterology* 1986;**90**:182–7.

59 Aarns PA, Branch RA. Prescribing for patients with liver disease. *Baillière's Clin Gastroenterol* 1989;**3**:109–30.

60 Westphal J-F, Brogard J-M. Drug administration in chronic liver diseases. *Drug Saf* 1997;**17**:47–73.

6: Heart failure

CATHERINE O'MALLEY, DERMOT PHELAN

Acute and chronic cardiac dysfunction

Acute cardiac failure, frequently superimposed on chronic cardiac impairment, is an everyday facet of critical illness. Indeed, cardiac dysfunction and sepsis – one of the causes of acute cardiac dysfunction – are the commonest causes of death in the intensive care unit (ICU).[1] The causes of multi-organ dysfunction syndrome (MODS) are varied and include hypovolaemia, sepsis, and the triggers of the systemic inflammatory response syndrome[2] such as pancreatitis, rhabdomyolysis, and postoperative massive transfusion. However, cardiac failure frequently contributes to organ dysfunction and it is standard practice to attempt to optimise cardiac function in an attempt to minimise or reverse organ dysfunction, for example, acute (pre-renal) renal impairment.

The average age of the adult critically ill patient population is 50–60 years, 30% are over 70 years old and the male to female ratio is 1·5:1.[1,3] In this group ischaemic heart disease, including previous myocardial infarctions, hypertensive, valvular, congenital, and cardiomyopathic heart disease, is common. Certain subpopulations, for example, cardiac and vascular surgery patients and general surgical patients admitted specifically because of known increased cardiac risk, increase the tendency to concentrate heart disease in the ICU. Diabetic patients and smokers, carrying an increased risk of cardiovascular disease including chronic obstructive pulmonary disease and right heart failure, constitute a disproportionate percentage of elective major surgery and ICU patients. Emergency postoperative admissions account for 23% of ICU patients[3] and carry much cardiovascular comorbidity related to cigarette smoking, alcohol abuse, and social and nutritional deprivation. Accompanying drug therapy such as ACE inhibitors, β-blockers, calcium antagonists, platelet antagonists, digoxin, diuretics, and bronchodilators add complexity to the acute illness both directly and by virtue of the interactions of the acute illness.

Pharmacokinetics in cardiac failure

Cardiac failure and its attendant multiple organ effects have variable influences on pharmacokinetic processes. It is important to note that many of the studies on the pharmacokinetic alterations in heart failure have been performed in patients with chronic and often stable disease, and many are small, with few patients, and are neither controlled nor randomised. In the critically ill patient, especially in the context of multiple organ dysfunction (MODS) or in the postoperative patient, it is difficult to isolate and interpret the clinical impact of cardiac failure on drug pharmacokinetics. Furthermore, concurrent therapies may be multiple, particularly in the ICU, and these may influence drug absorption, distribution, and elimination as well as receptor function. Nevertheless, an outline of some of the available information regarding the possible pharmacokinetic changes associated with cardiac failure may help to guide rational drug therapy in this patient population in the intensive care unit. These changes are summarised in Figure 6.1.

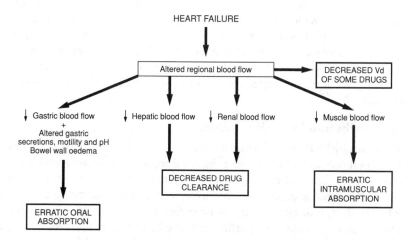

Figure 6.1   Pharmacokinetic changes in heart failure. Vd: Volume of distribution.

Drug absorption in cardiac failure

Drugs are usually given intravenously to the critically ill patient as this route is generally readily available and guarantees 100% bioavailability. If other routes of drug delivery are being contemplated, the influence of cardiac failure on drug absorption should be considered.

Cardiac failure may limit gastrointestinal absorption by several mechanisms. Decreased splanchnic blood flow, bowel wall oedema, alterations in gastric pH and secretions, and changes in gastrointestinal motility have all been implicated.[4] Furthermore, the routine of administration of medications such as morphine may impede gastric emptying and delay absorption.

Available data indicates impaired absorption of disopyramide,[5] quinidine,[6] hydrochlorothiazide,[7] and prazosin[8] in patients with cardiac failure.

103

Similarly, attainment of peak plasma concentrations of the phosphodi-esterase inhibitors milrinone and enoximone may be delayed due to slowed absorption.[9] By contrast, digoxin absorption appears to be unaltered in either right[10] or left heart failure.[11] The absorption of frusemide may be impaired in cardiac failure,[12 13] but there appears to be wide inter- and intra-patient variability.

Absorption of drugs following intramuscular injection is erratic. Even in healthy individuals variations in regional muscle blood flow result in differ-ent rates of absorption depending on the site of administration.[14] In patients with low cardiac output, blood flow to all muscle groups is decreased, ren-dering absorption more unpredictable. If an intramuscular injection is given during an episode of severe cardiovascular failure, where muscle blood sup-ply is markedly diminished, restoration of circulation may cause a delayed (but rapid) and potentially dangerous rise in blood concentration of the administered medication.[15] Lowered blood flow also renders muscle more prone to necrosis, which may complicate repeated intramuscular injections.

Multiple factors may influence drug absorption, particularly in the pres-ence of circulatory instability. Therefore, in critically ill patients with vari-able degrees of acute and chronic cardiac dysfunction, the enteral and intramuscular routes of drug administration are unreliable and may even be hazardous.

Drug distribution in cardiac failure

Of the multiple factors that influence drug distribution, cardiac output and regional blood flow are among the most important. In association with cardiac dysfunction, sympathetic nervous system activation and the admin-istration of certain exogenous catecholamines cause a decrease in blood flow to the liver, kidneys, and the peripheries in proportion to diminishing cardiac output.[16] Meanwhile, perfusion of the heart and brain is maintained by autoregulation and these organs may receive a disproportionate fraction of available cardiac output. The rate of drug distribution to regions of low-ered blood flow is therefore diminished with a subsequent decrease in vol-ume of distribution. The serum concentration of drugs which are normally rapidly distributed to the peripheral tissues, for example lignocaine, is increased.[17] Higher serum drug levels in combination with preferential flow to the heart and brain means that these organs are presented with a greater than normal drug concentration in cardiac failure. The myocardium and central nervous system are then more susceptible not only to the therapeu-tic but also the toxic effects of drugs that act at these sites. A single dose of lignocaine rapidly administered during acute cardiac failure has been reported to cause seizures.[18] By contrast, the distribution volume of drugs such as digoxin, which distribute slowly to the peripheral tissues, is largely unaltered in cardiac failure.

It has been suggested that the fluid accumulation in heart failure is asso-ciated with an increase in volume of distribution.[19] The weight of evidence suggests that this fluid is not in communication with the central vascular compartment and so does not contribute to central volume of distribution.[20] The volume of distribution of drugs such as frusemide,[4 13] theophylline,[21 22] midazolam,[23] and procainamide[24] is unchanged whilst that of quinidine[6] and paracetomol[25] is decreased.

The clinical implication of alterations in volume of distribution depends on the therapeutic range of the drug in question and on other factors, such as alterations in drug clearance. In general, loading doses, infusion rates, or maintenance doses of drugs with potential cardiotoxic and neurotoxic effects, whose distribution volume is diminished in cardiac failure, should be decreased and titrated carefully to effect. This is important, particularly when clearance is also decreased. Where appropriate, blood levels should be monitored. This would seem to be especially relevant during acute cardiac decompensation when alterations in blood flow and drug distribution may be at their most extreme.

Drug protein binding in cardiac failure

The clinical significance of alterations in the plasma protein binding of drugs is due to the resultant changes in concentration of the free, pharmacologically active form of the drug. Severe chronic congestive cardiac failure in the presence of normal serum protein content does not have any significant impact on the protein binding of digitoxin, phenytoin, diazepam, warfarin, propanolol, or imipramine.[26] This group is broadly representative of acidic, basic, and neutral compounds with both high and low degrees of ionisation as well as medications with high and low extraction ratios. These data suggest that the protein binding of many drugs is unaffected by cardiac failure alone.

However, hypoalbuminaemia may arise in cardiac failure caused by leakage into the interstitial fluid, diminished uptake, and impaired hepatic synthesis and drug protein binding may be reduced in heart failure by endogenous binding inhibitors such as free fatty acids and by metabolic acidosis.[27] In the ICU cardiac failure may be associated with the acute phase response or the systemic inflammatory response syndrome which are associated with hypoalbuminaemia and other protein abnormalities such as raised α_1-acid glycoprotein levels.

The limited evidence at hand suggests that the influence of cardiac failure on drug protein binding is probably clinically insignificant unless protein concentrations are altered. However, changes in drug protein binding cannot be ruled out, particularly when cardiac dysfunction occurs in the context of critical illness (see Figure 6.2).

Renal drug clearance in cardiac failure

Renal elimination is the principal route of clearance of many drugs and drug metabolites. Glomerular filtration, active tubular secretion, and passive tubular reabsorption, alone or in combination contribute to net drug excretion by the kidney. Cardiac failure may affect these key processes and thereby hinder renal drug handling.

105

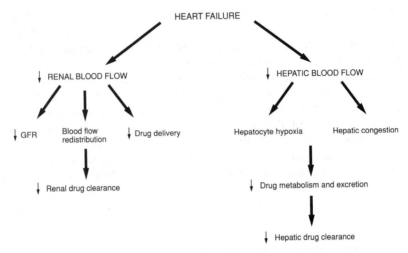

Figure 6.2 Altered drug clearance in heart failure. GFR: Glomerular filtration rate.

Normally the kidney receives 20% of cardiac output. In mild to moderate heart failure, increased renal vascular resistance causes a diminution of renal blood flow but autoregulation preserves glomerular filtration rate. In general, renal blood flow may decline chronically by 30–40% without apparent impairment of function. With progression of heart failure, however, decreased cardiac output and redistribution of blood flow away from the kidney eventually impinges on renal function. Afferent arteriolar vasoconstriction and a decrease in glomerular filtration rate occur. In cardiogenic shock flow declines to less than 15% of normal with medullary diversion, impairment of tubular function, and abnormal membrane transport secondary to diminished cellular oxygen delivery.[28]

Decreased glomerular filtration rate in heart failure may cause diminished clearance of drugs that are normally eliminated by this process. Tubular reabsorption of drugs may be increased due to redistribution of blood flow. Also, reduction in drug delivery rate ensuing from decreased perfusion can impair secretion. Drugs with high clearance, dependent on blood flow, are more affected by the changes brought about by cardiac failure than those which are cleared simply by glomerular filtration.[14]

Although cardiac failure may impair renal drug handling, the clinical significance of this effect in the presence of normal biochemical indices of renal function is unclear. Critically ill patients, however, may suffer from profound cardiac and circulatory disturbances with accompanying oliguria and azotaemia which may progress to fulminant renal failure and consequently impaired drug elimination. Inotropes and vasodilators, commonly employed in the treatment of critically ill patients, have variable effects on renal blood flow in patients with acute and chronic heart dysfunction. These may be due to direct effects on renal vascular resistance, intrarenal blood flow distribution or caused by alterations in cardiac output. The significance of each of these individual factors in the production of natriuresis, diuresis, and apparent improvement in renal function is controversial.

Creatinine clearance is traditionally used as a marker of the excretory capacity of the kidney. As alterations in drug clearance are presumed to be proportional to changes in creatinine clearance,[29] administration of drugs that undergo renal excretion to critically ill patients with cardiac failure should be guided by renal function. Therapeutic drug monitoring should be employed for drugs with a low therapeutic ratio, such as digoxin.

Hepatic drug clearance in cardiac failure

The liver is a vital organ of drug elimination and any condition that impairs hepatic function can potentially have an adverse effect on drug handling. Cardiac failure can cause hepatic impairment and consequently alter hepatic drug clearance. There are three factors commonly implicated in the pathogenesis of liver dysfunction caused by cardiac failure.[30] First, hepatocytes are extremely sensitive to hypoxia and arterial hypoxaemia may, in isolation, result in liver function test abnormalities. Heart failure is associated with peripheral venous hypertension and consequent passive congestion and oedema of the liver. Finally, the low output state of cardiac failure is associated with a proportionate diminution in blood flow to the liver.[16] The latter effect is associated with diminished clearance of drugs such as lignocaine[31] and the thrombolytic agent tissue plasminogen activator.[32]

The spectrum of the clinical and biochemical manifestations of hepatic dysfunction caused by cardiac failure is broad. Liver function tests may be only mildly abnormal and return to normal with treatment of the underlying condition. Occasionally abnormalities may persist for years,[33] for example, after heart transplantation.[34] In the cardiac intensive care unit, heart failure and accompanying hypotension resulting, for example, from cardiac tamponade, may give rise to the syndrome of ischaemic hepatitis. This condition, characterised by centrilobular hepatic necrosis, grossly elevated serum transaminases, and often accompanied by jaundice, is associated with high mortality.[35] The diminution in cardiac output and consequent decrease in liver blood flow impairs elimination of drugs with high extraction ratios. In one retrospective analysis, mortality in patients with ischaemic hepatitis was associated with a history of treatment with calcium channel blockers and antiarrhythmics. Diminished clearance of these potentially cardiodepressant drugs, pedisposing to toxicity, was believed to contribute to death.[36]

Whilst heart failure can result in demonstrable and occasionally severe abnormalities of liver function, there is no direct correlation between biochemical tests of liver function and the ability of the liver to metabolise drugs. In fact, abnormal drug handling occurs in the absence of overt, severe hepatic dysfunction. Model drugs such as aminopyrine and antipyrine, whose metabolism is well defined, have been used to demonstrate that the function of hepatic microsomal enzyme systems is impaired in heart failure. Diminished clearance of these drugs has been demonstrated in patients with congestive cardiac failure but normal or near-normal biochemical indices.[19][37][38] This impaired metabolic capacity and consequent decreased drug clearance is caused by the hepatocyte hypoxia and hepatic congestion associated with heart failure. The clearance of medications with low hepatic extraction ratios for example, theophylline, may be decreased in the presence of cardiac failure by this mechanism.[20][22]

Treatment of congestive cardiac failure results in lower venous pressures and an increase in cardiac index with a resultant decrease in centrilobular congestion and improved oxygenation of liver parenchyma. It might be expected that treatment of cardiac failure would bring about a correction of abnormal drug metabolism and clearance. This may not always be the case. In patients with severe cardiac failure refractory to other drugs, treatment with oral milrinone appears to improve hepatic metabolic function, reflected by aminopyrine metabolism. However, treatment with amrinone further diminishes metabolic activity. The reasons for this are unclear. As both drugs improve cardiac index and decrease right atrial pressure, it might be explained by an inhibitory effect of amrinone metabolites on the cytochrome P450 system or by effects on absorption.[38] Therefore, not only the presence of cardiac failure but also the effects of drugs used in its treatment may alter hepatic drug handling. Dopamine appears to have little or no effect on hepatic blood flow in adults with cardiac failure.[39] However, in children, following surgical repair of congenital heart lesions associated with preoperative heart failure, infusion of dopamine was shown to improve liver blood flow. The authors suggested that dopamine might exert a protective effect and minimise loss in liver function.[40] Whether or not this translates into improved drug clearance has not been studied.

Other vasodilator, vasopressor, and inotropic drugs used in the management of patients with cardiac failure have variable effects on liver blood flow (see Table 6.1). Evidence is scant with regard to their effects on clearance of

Table 6.1 The effect of vasoactive drugs on hepatic blood flow in cardiac failure.

Drug	Effect on hepatic blood flow in cardiac failure
Dopamine	Little effect on hepatic vascular resistance on hepatic blood flow[39]
Enoximone Milrinone Nitrates Nitroprusside Nifedipine Hydralazine	
Captopril Enalapril	Little effect or slight decrease in hepatic blood flow[39]
α_1-Adrenergic blockers Dopexamine	Increased hepatic blood flow[39]
Noradrenaline	Decreased hepatic blood flow[39]

drugs with either high or low extraction ratios. However, one animal study has shown that noradrenaline decreases the clearance of lignocaine by decreasing hepatic blood flow whereas isoprenaline increases lignocaine clearance by 40%.[17] Augmentation of cardiac output in end-stage cardiac failure by mechanical means may improve peripheral organ perfusion, including liver blood flow,[41] but the effect on drug clearance is not known.

It is clear that the effects of heart failure and its treatment on liver function are highly variable. Furthermore, the consequent alterations in drug metabolism and clearance may not be entirely predictable and restoration of normal cardiac function may not necessarily reverse derangements of hepatic function.

Changes of cardiac receptors with heart failure

Heart failure is associated with changes in the expression and function of several myocardial receptor populations, although patterns may vary according to the cause of the cardiac dysfunction. Understanding these changes allows better pharmacological therapy of heart failure.

There is a decrease in the cardiac β-adrenergic receptor number in the failing human heart, presumably owing to down-regulation in the face of chronic sympathetic nervous system activity.[42] As a consequence of the decrease in β-receptor density with cardiac failure, the contractile response to catecholamines is diminished, accounting for the insensitivity to exogenous catecholamines. Such down-regulation of β-receptors in donor hearts has been associated with fatal perioperative cardiac failure in heart transplant recipients.[43]

The extent of down-regulation correlates with the degree of failure,[44] whilst the relative density of β_1- and β_2-receptors varies according to cause. For example, in idiopathic dilated cardiomyopathy there is selective loss of β_1-receptors, while in mitral valve disease and ischaemic cardiomyopathy there is a concomitant reduction in β_1- and β_2-subtypes.[45] Furthermore, drug treatment affects β-receptor numbers. Calcium channel blockers appear to have no effect on β-receptor density while non-selective β-blockers are associated with up-regulation of both receptor subtypes.[46] The use of the selective β_1-antagonist metoprolol,[47] and the ACE inhibitor captopril[48] in heart failure cause an increase in β_1-receptor numbers. It seems possible that these effects may mediate some of the beneficial effects of β-blockers and ACE inhibitors alone, or in combination in the management of cardiac failure.

The effects of cardiac glycosides are mediated by inhibition of membrane-bound Na^+K^+ ATPase, the sodium pump. The positive inotropic effect of digoxin is the result of altered balance between intracellular sodium and calcium brought about by sodium pump blockade. The number of glycoside-binding sites is decreased in cardiac failure but certain isoforms of $Na^+ K^+$ ATPase are also diminshed in number and activity. Thus, blockade of functioning Na^+K^+ ATPase in the failing human heart further decreases activity and may account, in part, for the observed sensitivity to the inotropic effect of cardiac glycosides.[49]

The angiotensin I (AT-I) subpopulation of angiotensin receptors is down-regulated in cardiac failure and mediates the deleterious effects of angiotensin II in this condition.[50] These include myocyte hypertrophy, fibroblast proliferation, and vascular smooth muscle cell proliferation. Angiotensin II receptors are up-regulated in cardiac failure and appear to be anti AT-I in function, inhibiting collagen metabolism and the growth of cardiac fibroblasts in an animal model.[51] The benefits of ACE inhibitors in the secondary management of myocardial infarction and treatment of cardiac failure are well known. Direct AT-I receptor blockade may overcome some of the problems associated with ACE inhibitors, such as bradykinin-related side effects and lack of control of tissue angiotensin production. Furthermore, the beneficial effects of the two drug types may be additive; clinical studies are on-going.

Endothelin-1 is a coronary and peripheral vasoconstrictor contributing to increased vascular tone in severe, chronic heart failure[52] and exerts a concentration-dependent inotropic effect on failing human myocardium. The latter effect accounts for only 20–30% of that seen with maximal β-adrenergic receptor stimulation and is mediated by myocardial endothelin-A (ET-A) receptors which are up-regulated in cardiac failure. In a rat model, treatment with the selective ET-A receptor antagonist, bosentan, improved survival in association with improved cardiac output, decreased left ventricular hypertrophy and dilatation and cardiac fibrosis.[53] In humans, the short-term addition of bosentan to conventional therapy improved systemic and pulmonary haemodynamics in patients with severe chronic heart failure.[54] Longer-term benefits of ET-A receptor antagonists remain to be seen. These changes are summarised in Table 6.2

Table 6.2 Some of the changes in cardiac receptors.

Receptor	Effect	Result
β-Adrenoreceptor	Down-regulated	Catechoalmine insensitivity[44]
Digoxin receptor	Down-regulated	Enhanced inotropic effect[49]
AT-I receptor	Down-regulated	Myocyte hypertrophy, fibroblast proliferation, vascular smooth muscle cell proliferation[50]
AT-II receptor	Up-regulated	Inhibition of collagen metabolism, fibroblast growth[51]
ET-A receptor	Up-regulated	Coronary, peripheral vasoconstriction, inotropic effect[52]

Conclusion

Against the usual background of considerable chronic cardiovascular disease and therapies and the superimposition of critical illness with its plethora of acute cardiac dysfunctional effects, the bedside application of pharmacokinetic and pharmacodynamic principles will be complex in intensive care. Decisions regarding optimum cardiovascular therapy will also, in individual patients, be complex and unlikely to be amenable to predetermined formulae. Add to this the variety of direct effects of acute illness, especially septic and systemic inflammatory states, on pharmacokinetic factors such as volume of distribution and drug elimination and on pharmacodynamic factors such as receptor down-regulation and it is evident that cardiovascular therapy in the critically ill frequently needs moment by moment titration to effect and expert review. Although the choice of such titration strategies should obviously be scientifically based, there will be a large empirical element to practice with an emphasis on agreed clinical goals or end points.

As approximately 10% of hospital deaths among intensive care patients occur after patients leave ICU, it is probable that we should endeavour to avoid a hiatus in the continuity and intensity of care at the time of leaving ICU. The institution of step-down or high-dependency care may facilitate this but it is also likely that the transition from infused therapy to oral therapy should be recognised as a special risk period, particularly against a background of uncertain bioavailability, rapidly changing volume of distribution, and renal and hepatic elimination. Pharmacokinetic and pharmacodynamic drug interactions are also likely to occur. The need for care with transition from intravenous to oral therapy, for example, aminophylline to theophylline, hydrocortisone to prednisolone, esmolol to atenolol, and heparin to warfarin is readily accepted. This may entail a transition from perhaps a dobutamine infusion, mechanical intra-aortic balloon-pump support and mechanical ventilation to, say, digoxin and/or ACE inhibitors and/or diuretic therapy. Similar considerations apply to the early commencement or restarting of cardioprotective and antihypertensive therapies such as diltiazem and β-blockers when septic and high cardiac output and low blood pressure states are resolving.

1 Jordan DA, Miller CF, Kubos KL, Rogers MC. Evaluation of sepsis in a critically ill surgical population. *Crit Care Med* 1987;15:897–904.
2 Bone RC, Balk RA, Cerra FB *et al.* Definitions for sepsis and organ failure and guidelines for the use of innovative therapies in sepsis. The ACCP/SCCM Consensus Conference Committee. American College of Chest Physicians/Society of Critical Care Medicine. *Chest* 1992;101:1644–55.
3 Vincent JL, Bihari DJ, Suter P, *et al.* The prevalence of nosocomial infection in intensive care units in Europe. Results of the European Prevalence of Infection in Intensive Care (EPIC) Study. EPIC International Advisory Committee. *JAMA* 1995;274:639–44.
4 Benet LZ, Greither A, Meister W. Gastrointestinal absorption of drugs in patients with cardiac failure. In: Benet LZ, ed. *The effect of disease states on drug pharmacokinetics.* Washington DC: American Pharmaceutical Association, 1976.
5 Landmark K, Bredsen JE, Thaulow E, Simonsen S, Amlie JP. Pharmacokinetics of disopyramide in patients with imminent to moderate cardiac failure. *Eur J Clin Pharmacol* 1981;19:187–92.
6 Udea CT, Dzindzio BS. Bioavailability of quinidine in congestive heart failure. *Br J Clin Pharmacol* 1981;11:571–7.

7 Beermann B, Groschinsky-Grind M. Pharmacokinetics of hydrochlorothiazide in patients with congestive cardiac heart failure. *Br J Clin Pharmacol* 1979;7:579–83.

8 Baughman RA Jr, Arnold S, Benet LZ, Lin ET, Chatterjee K, Williams RL. Altered prazosin pharmacokinetics in congestive heart failure. *Eur J Clin Pharmacol* 1980;17:425–8.

9 Rocci ML, Wilson H. The pharmacokinetics and pharmacodynamics of newer inotropic agents. *Clin Pharmacokinet* 1987;13:91–109.

10 Ohnhaus EE, Vozeh S, Nuesch E. Absorption of digoxin in severe right heart failure. *Eur J Clin Pharmacol* 1979;15:115–20.

11 Meister W, Benowitz NL, Benet LZ. Unchanged absorption of digoxin tablets in patients with cardiac failure. *Pharmacology* 1984;28:90–4.

12 Vrhovac B, Sarapa N, Bakran I *et al.* Pharmacokinetic changes in patients with oedema. *Clin Pharmacokinet* 1995;28:405–18.

13 Vargo DL, Kramer WG, Black PK, Smith WB, Serpas T. Bioavailability, pharmacokinetics, and pharmacodynamics of torsemide and furosemide in patients with congestive heart failure. *Clin Pharmacol Ther* 1995;57:601–9.

14 Wilkinson GR. Pharmacokinetics in disease states modifying body perfusion. In: Benet LZ, ed. *The effect of disease states on drug pharmacokinetics*. Washington DC: American Pharmaceutical Association, 1976.

15 Pentel P, Benowitz N. Pharmacokinetic and pharmacodynamic considerations in drug therapy of cardiac emergencies. *Clin Pharmacokinet* 1984;9:273–308.

16 Leithe ME, Margorien RD, Hermiller JB, Unverferth DV, Leier CV. Relationship between central haemodynamics and regional blood flow in normal subjects and in patients with congestive heart failure. *Circulation* 1984;1:57–64.

17 Benowitz N, Forsyth RP, Melmon KL, Rowland M. Lidocaine disposition kinetics in monkey and man. II. Effects of haemorrhage and sympathomimetic drug administration. *Clin Pharmacol Ther* 1974;16:99–109.

18 Benowitz NL, Meister W. Clinical pharmacokinetics of lignocaine. *Clinical Pharmacokinet* 1978;3:177–201.

19 Hepner G, Vesell E, Tantum K. Reduced drug elimination in congestive heart failure studies using aminopyrine as a model drug. *Am J Med* 1978;65:271–6.

20 Shammas FV, Dickstein K. Clinical pharmacokinetics in heart failure. An updated review. *Clin Pharmacokinet* 1988;15:94–113.

21 Piafsky KM, Sitar DS, Rangno RE, Ogilvie RI. Theophylline kinetics in acute pulmonary oedema. *Clin Pharmacol Ther* 1977;21:310–16.

22 Uneo K, Miyai K, Koyama M, Seki T, Kawaguchi Y, Horiuchi Y. Effect of congestive heart failure on theophylline disposition. *Clin Pharmacol* 1990;9:936–7.

23 Patel IH, Soni PP, Fukuda EK, Smith DF, Leier CV, Boudoulas H. The pharmacokinetics of midazolam in patients with congestive heart failure. *Br J Clin Pharmacol* 1990;29:565–9.

24 Kessler KM, Kayden DS, Estes DM. Procainamide pharmacokinetics in patients with acute myocardial infarction or congestive heart failure. *J Am Coll Cardiol* 1986;7:1131–9.

25 Ochs HR, Schuppan U, Greenblatt DJ, Abernethy DR. Reduced distribution and clearence of acetaminophen in patients with congestive cardiac failure. *J Cardiovasc Pharmacol* 1983;5:697–9.

26 Fichtl B, Meister W, Schmied R. Serum protein binding of drugs is not altered in patients with severe congestive cardiac failure. *Int J Clin Pharmacol Ther Toxicol* 1983;21:241–4.

27 Tillement JD, Lhoste F, Giudicelli JF. Diseases and drug protein binding. *Clin Pharmacokinet* 1978;3:144–54.

28 Leier CV, Boudoulas H. Renal disorders and the heart. In: Braumwald E, ed. *Heart disease: a textbook of cardiovascular medicine*, 5th edn. Philadelphia: WB Saunders, 1997 : 1914.

29 Lam YWF, Banjerji S, Hatfield C, Talbert RL. Principles of drug administration in renal insufficiency. *Clin Pharmacokinet* 1997;32:30–57.

30 Holdstock G, Millward-Sadler GH, Wright R. Hepatic changes in systemic disease. In: Wright R, Millward-Sadler GH, Alberti KGMM, Karran S, eds. *Liver and biliary disease*, 2nd edn. London: Baillière Tindall, 1985 : 1049.

31 Prescott LF, Adjepon-Yamoah KK, Talbot RG. Impaired lignocaine metabolism in patients with myocardial infarction and cardiac failure. *BMJ* 1976;1:939–41.

32 van Griensven JM, Koster RW, Burggraaf J *et al.* Effects of liver blood flow on the pharmacokinetics of tissue plasminogen activator (alteplase) during thrombolysis in patients with acute myocardial infarction. *Clin Pharmacol Ther* 1998;63:39–47.

33 Cohen CD, Kirsch RE, Saunders SJ, Terblanche J. Hepatic sequelae of congestive cardiac

failure. Evidence for a liver lesion in patients in whom cardiac function has been restored to normal. *S Afr Med J* 1981;**14**:213–16.

34 Canderel JF, Grippon P, Mattie MF *et al.* Prevalence and causes of long-lasting hepatic dysfunction after heart transplantation: a series if 80 patients. *Artif Organs* 1988;**2**:234–8.

35 Gitlin N, Serio KM. Ischaemic hepatitis: widening horizons. *Am J Gastroenterol* 1992;**87**:831–6.

36 Potter JM, Hickman PE. Cardiodepressant drugs and the high mortality rate with ischaemic hepatitis. *Crit Care Med* 1992;**20**:474–8.

37 Manzione NC, Goldfarb JP, LeJemtel TH, Maskin CS, Sternlieb I. The effects of two new inotropic agents on microsomal liver function in patients with congestive heart failure. *Am J Med Sci* 1986;**291**:88–92.

38 Rissam HS, Nair CR, Anand IS, Madappa C, Wahi PI. Alteration of hepatic drug metabolism in female patients with congestive cardiac failure. *Int J Clin Pharmacol Ther Toxicol* 1983;**21**:602–4.

39 Leier CV. Regional blood flow responses to vasodilators and inotropes in congestive heart failure. *Am J Cardiol* 1988;**62**:86E–93E.

40 Mitchell IM, Pollock JC, Jamieson MP. Effects of dopamine on liver blood flow in children with congenital heart disease. *Ann Thorac Surg* 1995;**60**:1741–4.

41 Baldwin RT, Radovancevic B, Conger JL *et al.* Peripheral organ perfusion augmentation during left ventricular failure. A controlled bovine comparison between the intraaortic balloon pump and the hemopump. *Tex Heart Inst J* 1993;**20**:275–80.

42 Bristow MR, Lurie K, Ginsburg R *et al.* Decreased catecholamine sensitivity and beta-adrenergic receptor density in failing human hearts. *N Engl J Med* 1982;**307**:205–11.

43 Chester MR, Amadi AA, Barnett DB. Beta adrenoreceptor density in the donor heart: a guide to prognosis. *Br Heart J* 1995;**73**:540–1.

44 Steinfath M, Lavicky J, Schmitz W, Scholz H. Changes in cardiac beta adrenoreceptors in human heart disease and the relationship to the degree of heart failure and further evidence for etiology-related regulation of beta 1 and beta 2 subtypes. *J Cardiothorac Vasc Anesth* 1993;**7**:668–73.

45 Brodde OE, Zerkowski HR, Borst HG, Maier W, Michel MC. Drug- and disease-induced changes of human beta-1 and beta-2 adrenoreceptors. *Eur Heart J* 1989;**10**(Suppl B):38–44.

46 Jones CR, Fandeleur P, Harris B, Buhler FR. Effect of calcium and beta-adrenoreceptor antagonists on beta-adrenoreceptor density and Gs alpha expression in human atria. *Br J Clin Pharmacol* 1990;**30**:S171–3.

47 Sigmund M, Jakob H, Becker H *et al.* Effects of metoprolol on myocardial beta-adrenoreceptor and Gi alpha proteins in patients with congestive heart failure. *Eur J Clin Pharmacol* 1996;**51**:127–32.

48 Jakob H, Sigmund M, Eschenhagen T *et al.* Effect of captopril on myocardial beta-adrenoreceptor density and Gi alpha proteins I patients with mild to moderate heart failure and dilated cardiomyopathy. *Eur J Clin Pharmacol* 1995;**47**:389–94.

49 Schwinger RHG, Wang J, Frank K *et al.* Reduced sodium pump 1, 3 and 1-isoform protein levels and Na⁺, K⁺-ATPase activity but unchanged Na–Ca exchanger protein levels in human heart failure. *Circulation* 1999;**99**:2105–12.

50 McEwen PE, Gray GA, Sherry L, Webb DJ, Kenyon CJ. Differential effects of angiotensin II on cardiac cell proliferation and intramyocardial perivascular fibrosis in vivo. *Circulation* 1998;**15**:2765–73.

51 Ohkubo K, Matsubara H, Nozawa Y *et al.* Angiotensin type 2 receptors are reexpressed by cardiac fibroblasts from failing myopathic hamster hearts and inhibit cell growth and fibrillar collagen metabolism. *Circulation* 1997;**96**:3954–62.

52 Kiowski W, Sutsch G, Hunziker P *et al.* Evidence for endothelin-1-mediated vasoconstriction in severe chronic heart failure. *Lancet* 1995;**346**:732–6.

53 Mulder P, Richard V, Bouchart F, Derumeaux G, Munter K, Thuillez C. Selective ETA receptor blockade prevents left ventricular remodelling and deterioration of cardiac function in experimental heart failure. *Cardiovasc Res* 1998;**39**:600–8.

54 Sutsch G, Kiowski W, Yan XW *et al.* Short-term endothelin receptor antagonist therapy in conventionally treated patients with symptomatic severe chronic heart failure. *Circulation* 1998;**24**:2262–8.

7: Gut failure

GEOFFREY J DOBB

Changes in gastrointestinal function are common during critical illness. In everyday language to be "sick" is applied to all illness, but it is also specific to the gut. The gut responds vigorously to physiological stimuli. Sympathetic stimulation and catecholamines divert blood flow away from the gut and induce nausea. Parasympathetic stimuli are associated with hypotension and diarrhoea.

During critical illness the most profound changes in gut function occur during shock and multiple organ failure (Table 7.1). Much of the information available is derived from experimental studies. The relevance of the models used and species differences must be taken into account when considering the potential clinical implications. The clinical studies also have important limitations. For example, total hepato-splanchnic blood flow (including hepatic artery flow) and oxygen consumption can be measured in clinical studies but gut blood flow and oxygen consumption in isolation is not estimated because of the difficulty of obtaining samples from the portal vein. Also, few studies directly address the effects of altered gut function on the pharmacology of the critically ill.

Many of the drugs used in treating critically ill patients are given parenterally. Nevertheless, when drugs can be given in an enteral formulation this is usually cheaper and may be associated with reduced side effects. The disadvantage is uncertainty about their absorption and availability of formulations suitable for administration through naso-enteric feeding tubes. Studies of bioavailability of drugs in critically ill patients are further

Table 7.1 Changes in gastrointestinal function during shock and multiple organ failure.

- Changes in gut blood flow and distribution
- Mucosal ischaemia
- Increased mucosal permeability
- Altered gastrointestinal secretion
- Reduced uptake of substances dependent on active transport
- Altered gut motility
- Effects of drugs given on gut blood flow
- Effects of drugs given on gut motility
- Effect of continuous enteral nutrition

114

complicated by altered excretion, metabolism, volume of distribution or protein binding.

Changes in gut blood flow and distribution

Gut blood flow can be measured experimentally but clinical studies are limited by the methods available. In practice, total splanchnic – intestinal and hepatic flow – can be estimated using the Fick principle. Marker substances have included indocyanine green,[1] galactose,[2] and sorbitol.[3] Attempts to estimate blood flow just to the intestine have used aminopyrine clearance[4] and clearance of inert gas or hydrogen.[5][6] In experimental studies radioactive microspheres[7] can be used to examine intestinal intramural blood flow. A more recent technique, laser-doppler flowmetry, measures the blood flow in gastric mucosal capillaries[8] but the gastric mucosa must be visualised by gastroscopy making the technique unsuitable for routine or continuous use.

The intestinal villi have a central arteriole which branches at the top with blood flowing back down the villus through subepithelial capillaries and venules. This forms a counter-current arrangement which maintains oxygenation at the base of the villus at the expense of the top. The extremities of the "hairpin" loops in this counter-current arrangement are sensitive to reduced perfusion pressure, even if villus blood flow is unchanged. Reduced blood flow velocity causes reduction in oxygen tension at the tip of the villi.[9] Hypotension or ischaemic injury causes lifting of cells at the top of villi and then, as the injury becomes more severe or prolonged, epithelial cells are lost from the sides of the villus until its core is exposed and it disintegrates, the pattern of injury being related to the vascular anatomy of the villus. Once adequate perfusion is restored villus repair can be rapid. In rats, for example, mucosal repair occurs after just 18 hours.[10]

These anatomical changes and alterations in mucosal blood flow would be expected to have significant effects on functional drug absorption and the effective surface available.

Mucosal ischaemia

Experimental studies have shown that shock caused by haemorrhage, burns, trauma, sepsis and other causes of severe systemic inflammatory responses can produce intestinal ischaemia.[11] Oxygen delivery to the gut can decrease to 30% of the control value during haemorrhagic shock while oxygen consumption is unchanged. Septic shock caused by peritonitis decreases gut blood flow to a much lesser extent but intestinal oxygen consumption increases. During both forms of shock mucosal ischaemia is reflected by a mucosal intracellular acidosis[12] and during peritonitis oxygen extraction and utilisation may also be impaired through effects of endotoxin on oxidative phosphorylation[13] further exacerbating mucosal acidosis. With increasing severity of mucosal and gut ischaemia progressive injury occurs (Figure 7.1).

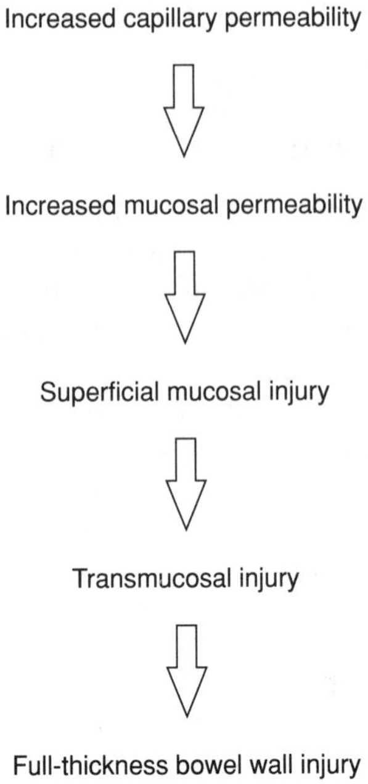

Increased capillary permeability

Increased mucosal permeability

Superficial mucosal injury

Transmucosal injury

Full-thickness bowel wall injury

Figure 7.1   Progression of injury caused by increasing mucosal and intestinal ischaemia.

Gastrointestinal lumenal tonometry provides an indication of relatively ischaemic intestinal mucosa, the assumption being that mucosal acidosis is caused by inadequate blood flow to meet the needs of mucosal cells.[14] While this technique does not provide any indication of absolute blood flow, it is logical to expect that acidotic mucosa will be dysfunctional and therefore that drug absorption may be affected. A study using laser-doppler flow-metry to assess mucosal blood flow supports the hypothesis that intramucosal acidosis is caused by gastric mucosal hypoperfusion[15] in mechanically ventilated patients. As yet, however, any association between mucosal acidosis and drug absorption has not been investigated.

Increased mucosal permeability

Differential absorption of non-metabolised substances has been used to assess mucosal permeability. Molecules used to assess mucosal permeability should be biologically inert, cross the mucosa by passive diffusion and be excreted in the urine to facilitate absorption after an oral dose. The proportion of the oral dose recovered, which provides the measure of permeability, will be affected by gastric emptying, intestinal transit and renal clearance. When using two molecules of different sizes, the non-mucosal confounding factors will apply to both so an increase in proportionate absorption of the larger molecule suggests increased mucosal permeability. Normally, the maximum channel size of the junctional complex between mucosal cells

116

allows molecules with a hydrodynamic molecular radius up to 1·1 mm to pass through. Lactulose and mannitol are commonly used because they are readily available and relatively easy to measure, but other substances including ethylene diamine tetra-acetic acid (EDTA), polyethylene glycol and L-rhamnose (thought to permeate transcellularly) have also been used.

Increased permeability has been shown in patients with haemorrhagic shock, trauma, sepsis, burns, and after major vascular surgery or cardiopulmonary bypass.[16-22] After cardiopulmonary bypass, increased gut permeability occurs independently of gastric mucosal acidosis assessed by tonometry, and there is no apparent relationship between the severity of gut ischaemia and permeability.[22] While this would appear to place in question the underlying role of gut ischaemia, other factors may play a role in increasing gut permeability in this setting, for example, cytokine activation during extracorporeal perfusion. Increases in intestinal permeability, as assessed by lactulose/mannitol ratios, are common in patients admitted to an intensive care unit[23], but a close relationship to illness severity or sepsis is not apparent.

Increased permeability might be expected to increase drug absorption, but any association between these two has yet to be demonstrated. In critically ill patients the effect of increased absorption related to increased permeability would be counteracted by decreased mucosal blood flow perhaps delaying uptake into the systemic circulation.

Altered gastrointestinal secretion

Shock, decreased intestinal blood flow, sympathomimetic drugs, and reduced or absent enteral nutrition reduce gastrointestinal secretion. Failure of gastric acid secretion is common in critically ill patients.[24] With reduced bicarbonate secretion into the proximal small bowel the normal pH changes occurring in the first part of the gut are altered and this will affect the absorption of pH-dependent drugs.

Most drugs are weak electrolytes so their absorption is affected by the pH of the intraluminal environment of the gut. They ionise to a greater or lesser extent according to the pH. In the non-ionised form drugs that are weak electrolytes are lipid soluble and diffusible whereas the ionised form is lipid insoluble and non-diffusible across cell membranes. Acidic groups are less ionised and basic groups more ionised in a low pH, and vice versa. Drugs that are highly ionised across the range of gut intraluminal pH are poorly or not absorbed by the enteral route. A few drugs (for example digoxin, chloramphenicol) do not ionise so their absorption is not affected by changes in intraluminal pH, though it can still be affected by changes in gut motility and loss of absorptive surface.

Reduced active transport

Differences between the absorption of molecules dependent on passive diffusion (see above) and substances dependent on active uptake, for example D-xylose and 3-o-methyl-D-glucose, provide a means of estimating the degree of active transport impairment associated with mucosal injury or changes in gut blood flow.[25] During sepsis the uptake of 3-o-methyl-D-glucose is greatly decreased compared to normal control values, the amount of absorption being inversely proportional to the patients' serum lactate concentration.[18] Shock reduces intestinal amino acid absorption[26], this persisting after resuscitation has restored both arterial pressure and splanchnic blood flow, suggesting delayed recovery of active amino acid transport by the mucosa. Gut lipid transport is impaired after trauma and haemorrhagic shock[27] and this appears to be caused, at least in part, by decreased intestinal alkaline phosphatase activity in the mucosal cells of the intestinal villi. Similar effects are probable on drugs dependent on active uptake.

Of interest, in experimental studies, some of the effects of shock on gut absorptive capacity are reversed by ATP-magnesium chloride, heparin or diltiazem,[28-30] but these effects have not been confirmed by clinical studies.

Altered gut motility

Impaired gastric emptying is common in critically ill patients[31] and very common in those with brain injury.[32] Migrating motor complexes originating from the antrum are inhibited by many of the factors associated with critical illness (Table 7.2). High sympathetic tone and catecholamine concentrations probably contribute to ileus by causing splanchnic hypoperfusion. For example, this appears to be the cause of ileus and other abdominal complications after cardiac surgery[33] and splanchnic ischaemia is common after isolated neurotrauma[34] when delayed gastric emptying is also common.

Usually the stomach does not have a major role in drug absorption, even for acidic drugs that are non-ionised and lipid-soluble at normal gastric pH, because the surface area is very much smaller than that of the small intestine and gastric emptying is relatively fast (half-time for gastric emptying approximately 30 minutes). However, reduced gastric acidity (see above), delayed

Table 7.2   Factors affecting gut motility.

- Peritonitis
- Intestinal ischaemia
- Retroperitoneal haemorrhage
- Laparotomy
- Bowel banding or surgery
- Trauma
- General or spinal anaesthesia
- Spinal cord lesion
- Hypothyroidism
- Electrolyte abnormalities
- Drugs: narcotic analgesics, phenothiazines, tricyclic antidepressants, calcium antagonists, etc.
- High sympathetic tone

gastric emptying, and loss of effective absorptive surface from the small intestine may alter the absorption of drugs in ways that are difficult to predict.

Effect of drugs on gut blood flow

After fluid resuscitation, intestinal perfusion partly recovers[35] and may cause reperfusion injury with activation of inflammatory mediators.[11] The effects of sympathiomimetics that may be used to support the circulation have been less marked than expected in experimental models. For example, dobutamine, dopamine, dopexamine and noradrenaline have no significant effect on stomach, small or large intestine blood flow in sheep[36] even though all increase cardiac output. In septic sheep the circulation is less sensitive to the effects of sympathomimetics.

There may, however, be some interspecies difference because clinical studies in critically ill patients have shown differences between the effects of sympathomimetics in their effects on mucosal ischaemia, at least as assessed by gastric tonometry. Dopamine increased gastric mucosal acidosis in patients with hyperdynamic sepsis when used to maintain a mean arterial pressure greater than 75 mmHg, whereas noradrenaline used to maintain the same arterial pressure decreased mucosal acidosis.[37]

In patients with septic shock, who had already had fluid resuscitation and dopamine 20 micrograms/kg/min, a randomised comparison of adrenaline versus a combination of noradrenaline and dobutamine[38] found adrenaline tended to worsen gastric mucosal acidosis, whereas noradrenaline–dobutamine tended to return mucosal pH towards normal. In another small study of six patients with hyperdynamic septic shock,[39] replacing noradrenaline with phenylephrine reduced splanchnic blood flow and oxygen delivery without affecting systemic haemodynamics or splanchnic oxygen consumption. It therefore appeared that, at least under the study's conditions, exogenous β-adrenergic stimulation was an important determinant of splanchnic blood flow.

Some potential insight into the apparently variable effects of low dose dopamine on splanchnic blood flow is provided by a prospective controlled trial[40] in which dopamine 3 micrograms/kg/min increased splanchnic blood flow, and also splanchnic oxygen consumption, in patients with septic shock and a low fractional splanchnic blood flow (less than 30% of cardiac output), but had no effect when splanchnic blood flow was greater than 30% of the total. Redistribution of blood flow within the bowel, with diversion away from the mucosa, might also account for some of the investigational findings.

A review[41] of clinical and experimental studies of the effects of vasoactive agents on gastric intramucosal pH concludes that the effects are unpredictable. While, of the catecholamines, dopamine was the least likely and dobutamine the most likely to increase mucosal pH. Noradrenaline generally increased the pH, adrenaline decreased it and the information available on dopexamine, nitric oxide donors and blockers, pentoxifylline and N-acetylcysteine was insufficient to reach a conclusion. This review omitted

119

consideration of angiotensin-converting enzyme (ACE) inhibitors. Although these are very rarely introduced in critically ill or shocked patients, it is known that angiotensin is a potent splanchnic vasoconstrictor and many patients with hypertension or cardiac failure receive long term treatment with ACE inhibitors. Most of those widely used now are long-acting. In an experimental study[42] enalapril prevented the reduction in splanchnic oxygen delivery induced by acute hypovolaemia and maintained duodenal function. The angiotensin II type 1 receptor antagonist losartan improved gut oxygen delivery after an endotoxin challenge but did not prevent ileal mucosal acidosis.[43] The clinical relevance of these studies has still to be confirmed and the benefit of supporting gut blood flow at the potential expense of other organs is unclear.

The implications of the effects of drugs used in critically ill patients for drug absorption from the gut are untested, though clearly mucosal blood flow has a role in drug absorption and mucosal acidosis will affect the uptake of partially ionised agents.

Effect of drugs on gut motility

Cisapride,[31 44] metoclopramide[45] and erthyromycin[46] can increase the rate of gastric emptying in critically ill patients and will therefore tend to accelerate drug absorption. Paracetamol, which is only absorbed effectively after leaving the stomach, has been used in many studies to assess gastric emptying. In a study of 27 intensive care unit patients, the area under the plasma concentration curve for paracetamol between zero and 60 minutes (AUC 60) after intragastric administration varied widely between the different patients.[47] Although there was an association between the AUC 60 and patients' risk of death predicted from their severity of illness (APACHE II score 24 hours before the study), this was weak with $r^2 = 0.25$. Of interest, low dose dopamine 2·5–5 micrograms/kg/min was associated with a significantly decreased mean rate of gastric emptying, but this finding has still to be confirmed.

Many of the drugs used for analgesia and sedation, and those with cholinergic effects, reduce gut motility.

Effect of continuous enteral nutrition

Many critically ill patients receive nutritional support by continuous enteral feeding. While some have advocated the use of intermittent feeds, the intragastric pH in this patient population tends to be similar whether feeds are given continuously or intermittently[48,49] so gastric pH should not be a major factor affecting drug absorption. However, it is known that the absorption of some drugs, for example phenytoin, is reduced when given with enteral feeds. In general, if the product information provided with a drug recommends that it be taken with an empty stomach, enteral feeding is preferably stopped for a period before and after its administration. With phenytoin, for example, we have found stopping the feeds for two hours before and one hour after the dose enhances absorption and facilitates obtaining stable plasma concentrations. Concurrent enteral feeding has also been observed to slow the absorption of carbamazepine.[50]

Nevertheless, the enteral route remains an option, even in critically ill patients, and some drugs can be surprisingly well absorbed. For example, a case report[51] confirms that oral ciprofloxacin can be well absorbed even in the presence of cardiogenic shock and multiple organ failure.

The major problem is uncertainty about enteral absorption and the limited information available about the effect of factors such as continuous enteral feeding on drug absorption. An additional difficulty is the lack of suitable formulations of many drugs. Relatively few are available as elixirs or suspensions.

Feeding tube obstruction by medications is one of the most common complications of enteral nutrition.[52] This is because medications are often crushed before they are flushed down the tube with some of the particles remaining too large to pass easily. Crushing tablets may also alter their absorption characteristics, with solutions and suspensions usually being absorbed more rapidly than capsules or tablets. Clearly some preparations, such as enteric coated tablets or sustained release formulations, are not designed for crushing though this may still occur because the implications are not understood.[52,53] Even with standard tablets, crushing will affect their disintegration and dissolution and therefore their potential bioavailability. These issues contribute to the relatively high adverse drug event rates in critically ill patients.[53,54]

Rectal administration

While some drugs are available as suppositories for rectal administration, few of those commonly needed by critically ill patients come in this form. Absorption of drugs from the rectum during critical illness is not well documented. The relatively high frequency of diarrhoea in patients needing intensive care[55] may also cause difficulty with this route.

Conclusion

Critically ill patients are often unable to swallow oral medications and many of the drugs needed are only available parenterally. Concerns regarding the oral absorption of important medications also inhibit enteral administration of drugs during intensive care. Complex interactions between the effects of severe illness on gut motility, blood flow and other factors affecting absorption also make predictions of bioavailability of drugs during the acute phase of a patient's illness uncertain. Substantial differences are likely between patients and within patients over time.

As a patient's condition improves, gut function also improves and enteral drug administration should be considered. Enteral formulations are usually

121

cheaper, but their suitability for giving through feeding tubes and potential interaction with continuous feeds should be assessed first.

The rectal route is an alternative which has been under-investigated and possibly under-used, but few drugs are available in a suitable formulation.

1 Caesar J, Shaldon S, Chiandussi L, Guevara L, Sherlock S. The use of indocyanine green in the measurement of hepatic blood flow and as a test of hepatic function. *Clin Sci* 1961;**21**:43–57.
2 Henderson JM, Kutner MH, Bain RP. First order clearance of plasma galactose: the effect of liver disease. *Gastroenterology* 1982;**83**:1090–6.
3 Zech J, Lange H, Bosch J, *et al.* Steady-state extrarenal sorbitol as a measure of hepatic plasma flow. *Gastroenterology* 1988;**95**:749–59.
4 Sack J, Spenney JG. Aminopyrine accumulation by mammalian gastric glands: an analysis of the technique. *Am J Physiol* 1982;**250**:G313–19.
5 Gharagozloo F, Bulkley GB, Zuidema GD, O'Mara CS, Alderson PO. The use of intraperitoneal xenon for early diagnosis of acute mesenteric ischemia. *Surgery* 1984;**95**:404–11.
6 Ashley SW, Cheung LY. Measurements of gastric mucosal blood flow by hydrogen gas clearance. *Am J Physiol* 1984;**247**:G339–45.
7 Dregelid E, Haukaas S, Amundsen S *et al.* Microsphere method in measurement of blood flow to wall layers of small intestine. *Am J Physiol* 1986;**250**:G670–78.
8 Kvietys PR, Sheperd AP, Granger DN. Laser-doppler, H_2 clearance, and microsphere estimates of mucosal blood flow. *Am J Physiol* 1985;**249**:G221–27.
9 Lundren O, Haglund U. The pathophysiology of the intestinal countercurrent exchanger. *Life Sci* 1978;**23**:1411–22.
10 Park PO, Haglund U. Regeneration of small bowel mucosa after intestinal ischaemia. *Crit Care Med* 1992;**20**:135–9.
11 Turnage RH, Guice KS, Oldham KT. Pulmonary microvascular injury following intestinal reperfusion. *New Horizons* 1994;**2**:463–75.
12 Antonsson JB, Haglund UH. Gut intramucosal pH and intraluminal Po_2 in a porcine model of peritonitis or haemorrhage. *Gut* 1995;**37**:791–7.
13 Schaefer CF, Biber B, Lerner MR, Jobis-Vandervliet FF, Fagraeus L. Rapid reduction of intestinal cytochrome-a, a^3 during lethal endotoxemia. *J Surg Res* 1991;**51**:382–91.
14 Gutierrez G, Brown SD. Gastrointestinal tonometry: a monitor of regional dysoxia. *New Horizons* 1996;**4**:413–19.
15 Elizalde JI, Hernandez C, Llach J *et al.* Gastric intramucosal acidosis in mechanically ventilated patients: role of mucosal blood flow. *Crit Care Med* 1998;**26**:827–32.
16 Roumen RMH, Hendriks, T, Wevers RA, Goris RJA. Intestinal permeability after severe trauma and hemorrhagic shock is increased without relation to septic complications. *Arch Surg* 1993;**128**:453–7.
17 Deitch EA, Berg R, Specian R. Endotoxin promotes the translocation of bacteria from the gut. *Arch Surg* 1987;**122**:185–90.
18 Johnson JD, Harvey CJ, Menzies IL, Treacher DF. Gastrointestinal permeability and absorptive capacity in sepsis. *Crit Care Med* 1996;**24**:1144–9.
19 LeVoyer T, Cioffi WG, Pratt L *et al.* Alteration in intestinal permeability after thermal injury. *Arch Surg* 1992;**127**:26–30.
20 Roumen RM, van der Vliet JA, Wevers RA, Goris RJ. Intestinal permeability is increased after major vascular surgery. *J Vasc Surg* 1993;**17**:734–7.
21 Ohri SK, Bjarnason I, Pathi V *et al.* Cardiopulmonary bypass impairs small intestinal transport and increases gut permeability. *Ann Thoracic Surg* 1993;**55**:1080–6.
22 Riddington DW, Venkatesh B, Boivin RS *et al.* Intestinal permeability, gastric intramucosal pH, and systemic endotoxemia in patients undergoing cardiopulmonary bypass. *JAMA* 1996;**275**:1007–12.
23 Harris CE, Griffiths RD, Freestone N, Billington D, Atherton ST, Macmillan RR. Intestinal permeability in the critically ill. *Intensive Care Med* 1992;**18**:38–41.
24 Stannard VA, Hutchinson A, Morris DL, Byrne A. Gastric exocrine "failure" in critically ill patients: incidence and associated features. *BMJ* 1988;**296**:155–6.
25 Travis S, Menzies I. Intestinal permability: functional assessment and significance. *Clin Sci* 1992;**82**:477–88.

26 Sodeyama M, Kirk SJ, Regan MC, Barbul A. The effect of hemorrhagic shock on intestinal amino acid absorption *in vivo*. *Circ Shock* 1992;**28**:153–6.

27 Wang W, Wang P, Chaudry IH. Intestinal alkaline phosphatase: role in the depressed gut lipid transport after trauma-hemorrhagic shock. *Shock* 1997;**8**:40–4.

28 Singh G, Chaudry KI, Chaudry IH. ATP-MgCl$_2$ restores gut absorptive capacity early after trauma-hemorrhagic shock. *Am J Physiol* 1993;**264**:R977–83.

29 Singh G, Chaudry KI, Chaudry IH. Restoration of gut absorptive capacity following trauma-hemorrhagic shock by the adjuvent use of heparin sulfate. *J Trauma* 1993;**34**:645–51.

30 Singh G, Chaudry KI, Chadler LC, Chaudry IH. Depressed gut absorptive capacity early after trauma-hemorrhagic shock. Restoration with diltiazem treatment. *Ann Surg* 1991;**214**:712–18.

31 Spapen HD, Duinslaeger L, Diltoer M, Gillet R, Bossuyt A, Huyghens LP. Gastric emptying in critically ill patients is accelerated by adding cisapride to a standard enteral feeding protocol: results of a prospective, randomised, controlled trial. *Crit Care Med* 1995;**23**:481–5.

32 Norton JA, Ott LG, McClain C *et al*. Intolerance to enteral feeding in the brain injured patient. *J Neurosurg* 1988;**68**:62–6.

33 Christenson JT, Schmuziger M, Maurice, Simonet F, Velebit V. Postoperative visceral hypotension: the common cause for gastrointestinal complications after cardiac surgery. *Thorac Cardiovasc Surg* 1994;**42**:152–7.

34 Venkatesh B, Townsend S, Boots RJ. Does splanchnic ischemia occur in isolated neurotrauma? A prospective observational study. *Crit Care Med* 1999;**27**:1175–80.

35 Scannell G, Clark L, Waxman K. Regional blood flow during experimental haemorrhage and crystalloid resuscitation: persistence of low flow to the splanchnic organs. *Resuscitation* 1992;**23**:217–25.

36 Bersten AD, Hersch M, Cheung H, Rutledge FS, Sibbald WJ. The effects of various sympathomimetics on the regional circulation in hyperdynamic sepsis. *Surgery* 1992;**112**:549–61.

37 Marik PE, Mohedin M. The contrasting effects of dopamine and norepinephrine on systemic and splanchnic oxygen utilisation in hyperdynamic sepsis. *JAMA* 1994;**272**:1254–357.

38 Levy B, Bollaert PE, Charpentier C *et al*. Comparison of norepinephrine and dobutamine to epinephrine for hemodynamics, lactate metabolism and gastric tonometric variables in septic shock: a prospective randomized study. *Intensive Care Med* 1997;**23**:282–7.

39 Reinelt H, Radermacher P, Kiefer P *et al*. Impact of exogenous beta-adrenergic receptor stimulation on hepato-splanchnic oxygen kinetics and metabolic activity in septic shock. *Crit Care Med* 1999;**27**:325–31.

40 Meier-Hellman A, Bredle DL, Specht M, Spies C, Hannemann L, Reinhart K. The effects of low-dose dopamine on splanchnic blood flow and oxygen uptake in patients with septic shock. *Intensive Care Med* 1997;**23**:31–7.

41 Silva E, DeBacker D, Creteur J, Vincent JL. Effects of vasoactive drugs on gastric intramucosal pH. *Crit Care Med* 1998;**26**:1749–58.

42 Aneman A, Pettersson A, Eisenhofer G *et al*. Sympathetic and renin-angiotensin activation during graded hypovolemia in pigs: impact on mesenteric perfusion and duodenal mucosal function. *Shock* 1997;**8**:378–84.

43 Oldner A, Wanecek M, Weitzberg E *et al*. Angiotensin II receptor antagonism increases gut oxygen delivery but fails to improve intestinal mucosal acidosis in procine endotoxin shock. *Shock* 1999;**11**:127–35.

44 Goldhill DR, Toner CC, Tarling MM, Baxter K, Withington PS, Whelpton R. Double-blind randomised study of the effect of cisapride on gastric emptying in critically ill patients. *Crit Care Med* 1997;**25**:447–51.

45 Jooste CA, Mustoe J, Collee G. Metoclopramide improves gastric motility in critically ill patients. *Intensive Care Med* 1999;**25**:464–8.

46 Dive A, Miesse C, Galanti L *et al*. Effect of erythromycin on gastric motility in mechanically ventilated critically ill patients: a double-blind, randomised, placebo-controlled study. *Crit Care Med* 1995;**23**:1356–62.

47 Tarling MM, Toner CC, Withington PS, Baxter MK, Whelpton R, Goldhill DR. A model of gastric emptying using paracetamol absorption in intensive care patients. *Intensive Care Med* 1997;**23**:256–60.

48 Bonten MJ, Gaillard CA, van der Hulst R *et al*. Intermittent enteral feeding: the influence

on respiratory and digestive tract colonisation in mechanically ventilated intensive care unit patients. *Am J Resp Crit Care Med* 1996;**154**:394–9.

49 Spilker CA, Hinthorn DR, Pingleton SK. Intermittent enteral feeding in mechanically ventilated patients. The effect on gastric pH and gastric cultures. *Chest* 1996;**110**:243–8.

50 Miles MV, Lawless ST, Tennison MB, Zaritsky AL, Greenwood RS. Rapid loading of critically ill patients with carbamazepine suspension. *Pediatrics* 1990;**86**:263–6.

51 Ujhelyi MR, Sullivan M, Nightingale C. Absorption of oral ciprofloxacin in a patient with cardiogenic shock. *Pharmacotherapy* 1991;**11**:336–9.

52 Belknap DC, Seifert CF, Peterman M. Administration of medications through enteral feeding catheters. *Am J Crit Care* 1997;**6**:382–92.

53 Cerulli J, Malone M. Assessment of drug-related problems in clinical nutrition patients. *JPEN* 1999;**23**:218–21.

54 Cullen DJ, Sweitzer BJ, Bates DW, Burdick E, Edmondson A, Leape LL. Preventable adverse drug events in hospitalised patients: a comparitive study of intensive care and general care units. *Crit Care Med* 1997;**25**:1289–97.

55 Ringel AF, Jameson GL, Foster ES. Diarrhea in the intensive care patient. *Crit Care Clinics* 1995;**11**:465–77.

8: Brain failure

JEAN-PIERRE MUSTAKI, BRUNO BISSONNETTE,
RENÉ CHIOLÉRO, ATUL SWAMI

Introduction

Over the last decade, there has been a rapid development of neuro-science. This includes the field of neurological critical care, where new therapeutic strategies and pharmacological agents have been proposed to manage patients with severe brain trauma, cerebrovascular disease, or refractory epilepsy. Similarly, a better understanding of brain physiology and pathophysiological mechanisms has stimulated the development of new concepts for brain protection.

The pharmacological approach to the patient with acute brain failure includes three main aspects:

1. When in the ICU, these patients have similar pharmacological require-ments to other critically ill patients in many aspects of their medical management. This is particularly true for treatments directed to systems other than the brain.
2. Specific treatments are prescribed for indications related to brain diseases (e.g. fibrinolysis in a patient with acute stroke) or to influence cerebral pathophysiological processes, like intracranial hypertension or cerebral ischaemia.
3. Other pharmacological treatments, without direct cerebral effect, may indirectly influence the brain function, via systemic effects, such as modifications of arterial blood pressure, cardiac output, blood gases, etc.

How brain failure changes the effects of these agents on normal and abnormal brains is the subject of this chapter. When prescribing any pharmacological agents to patients with acute brain failure, it is thus imper-ative to integrate the relevant neurological pathophysiological conditions to any changes that may be attributed to that drug. For example, before prescribing a vasodilator in order to reduce systemic vascular resistance (e.g. nitroglycerine, sodium nitroprusside, calcium antagonist, etc.), it is imperative to determine the actual condition of the cerebral circulation and the intracranial pressure (ICP) of the patient, as well as the expected effects of the different drugs on these variables.

Physiology and pathophysiology

Cerebral blood flow and perfusion

The adult brain has a very high cerebral blood flow related to its weight: in normal circumstances, cerebral blood flow (CBF) amounts to 750–850 ml/min (45–65 ml/min per 100 g tissue), corresponding to 15–20% of total cardiac output, while the brain weighs about 1·5 kg, or 2–3% of the total body weight. The cerebral metabolic oxygen consumption ($CMRO_2$) is also high, amounting to about 20% of body oxygen consumption (3·0–3·6 ml/min per 100 g). In normal circumstances there is a tight coupling between the CBF and cerebral metabolic rate (or $CMRO_2$). This flow–metabolic coupling is a complex phenomenon, probably related to local metabolic mechanisms.

Under normal circumstances, glucose is the main substrate for energy production since free fatty acids do not cross the blood–brain barrier and therefore do not constitute a substrate for energy metabolism in the brain. Each day, about 120 g glucose (4·8–5·5 ml/min per 100 g) is oxidised by brain cells. In neonates, as well as in adults, during prolonged starvation, ketone bodies may largely replace glucose for energy production.

It can be calculated that about 40% of the energy consumed by the brain is used to maintain the cellular membranes and the blood–brain barrier (BBB) integrity. The other 60% is used to generate electrical influxes and synthesise neurotransmitters. Owing to its high intrinsic oxygen consumption and to the absence of any significant oxygen reserve, the brain is highly sensitive to ischaemia and hypoxia. Any interruption of CBF exceeding 8–10 seconds leads to unconsciousness and eventually the development of coma. In most conditions, irreversible cellular injury occurs after 3–8 minutes, when ATP reserves and other energy producing mechanisms are exhausted. The sensitivity of various cerebral areas to hypoxia is not uniform: some areas, like the limbic system, Purkinje cells in the cerebellum and nerve layers of 3, 5 and 6 of the cerebral cortex, are particularly sensitive and prone to develop early injury.

The cerebral perfusion pressure (CPP) is dependent on both the levels of mean arterial blood pressure (MAP) and intracranial pressure: CPP = MAP – ICP. In a healthy subject, a CPP value ranging between 50–150 mmHg is adequate to ensure an adequate CBF, while levels below 50 mmHg lead to decreased CBF. When CBF decreases further below the ischaemic threshold (20–30 ml/min per 100 g), there is slowing of the EEG waves, followed by flattening and eventually the disappearance of cerebral electrical activity. This phenomenon, first reversible, becomes irreversible when cell death occurs.

In normal circumstances, CBF stays constant, despite wide fluctuations of MAP. This phenomenon, called cerebral autoregulation, is related to metabolic (adenosine, H^+, K^+ ions), myogenic and neurogenic mechanisms, and to other factors including nitric oxide (NO). This autoregulation requires a 30–120 second delay to be fully effective, during which acute changes in MAP induce parallel changes in CBF. In patients with altered autoregulation (brain injury, anoxia, haemorrhage, tumour, hypercapnia, hypoxemia, etc.), any marked haemodynamic instability may alter CBF in the diseased cerebral zone.[1]

Ischaemia

Cerebral ischaemia induces complex pathophysiological consequences, often called the ischaemic cascade. The critical reduction of CBF provokes a cascade of events which will further amplify the cellular consequences of ischaemia. Reperfusion, which follows transient ischaemia, also participates in the development of neuronal injury. It is characterised by a biphasic evolution: there is first a brief period of hyperaemia, followed by a more prolonged period of relative hypoperfusion. The reduction of energy production by the cell during ischaemia is associated with a switch to anaerobic metabolism, intracellular acidosis, and with a progressive alteration to the BBB. A few minutes after brain electrical activity stops, there is a progressive intracellular accumulation of both sodium and calcium ions. The resulting electrochemical depolarisation leads to the release of excitatory amino acids such as glutamate and aspartate, which promote calcium entry, lipid peroxidation, prostanoids and free radical formation. This provokes further injury to cell membranes and finally induces cell death.[2]

It is a well known clinical and laboratory phenomenon that hyperglycemia and increases in brain glucose worsen cerebral injury after a period of complete or near complete ischaemia. During ischaemia the brain anaerobically metabolises glucose to lactic acid. If the ischaemic insult occurs during a period of elevated brain glucose, lactic acid formation will be increased creating a pathological acidic intracellular environment. It appears that ischaemic brain lactate levels must increase to greater than 20 μmol/g to produce irreversible brain damage. The molecular basis by which the increased cellular acid load produces irreversible cell damage is unknown. Dextrose containing solutions are avoided since the residual free water can worsen cerebral oedema and because the associated elevations in blood sugar may worsen outcome.[3]

Cerebral blood volume, intracranial pressure

The adult brain is composed of 70–80% water, distributed in the intracellular, interstitial, cerebrospinal fluid and blood compartments. The remaining 20–30% includes several types of brain cells. The ICP depends on intracranial tissues and fluid components (CSF, blood) which are contained in a rigid cranial box. In normal conditions, ICP amounts to 0–15 mmHg. When the volume of one of these components increases, this may initially be compensated by a concomitant decrease in another component. However, when intracranial volume increases further, this induces a secondary rise of ICP, owing to the exhaustion of the compensatory mechanisms. The characteristic pressure–volume curve in three situations with different cerebral compliance is schematised in Figure 8.1. The curve

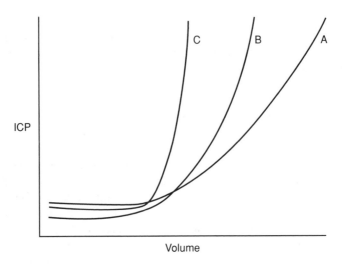

Figure 8.1   Schematic pressure/volume curves. A = normal cerebral compliance;
B: moderate cerebral compliance; C: low cerebral compliance.

clearly shows that when the intracranial content increases over a given value
(corresponding to the elbow of the pressure/volume (P/V) curve), there is a
rapid and disproportionate increase in ICP. This can occur with simple
stimuli, like coughing against the tracheal tube.[4]

Blood–brain barrier

Drugs have to cross the capillary endothelium to gain access into brain
tissue. In the brain, the capillary endothelium exerts a barrier function,
mainly related to the tight intercellular junctions. The specialised ependyma
of the circumventricular organs exerts similar barrier function. The high
electrical resistance of these membranes makes ion permeability very low:
diffusion across them requires an ATP-dependent pump system. Facilitated
transport exists for glucose, amino acids and several organic non-
electrolytes. Hormones, numerous drugs and other substances bound to
plasma proteins are delivered to sites of BBB where diffusion or carrier-
mediated transfer occurs. Vesicular transporters have been advocated as
another mechanism of transfer through cerebral endothelial cells. Transport
by CBF to the sites of transfer in the BBB can also modify patterns of
penetration for highly permeable drugs such as thiopental and nicotine,
which distribute during the first pass period (<10 seconds) to high flow
areas of the CNS. The diffusion of the unionised and unbound fraction of a
substance depends on its molecular weight, lipid solubility, electrical polarity and protein binding. Water diffusion obeys Starling forces, osmotic

128

action as well as tonicity and osmotic reflection. Practically, a large majority of ionised compounds (electrolytes, muscle relaxants), proteins and high molecular weight sugars (mannitol) do not cross the BBB in normal conditions, while glucose crosses readily through it. The BBB is relatively impermeable to water molecules. This contrasts with the microcirculation in muscle and viscera, where small particles like mannitol, electrolytes, and water, readily cross the capillary walls.[4]

Several conditions may alter BBB integrity and permeability: age,[5] hyperthermia,[6] traumatic injury,[7,8] arterial hypertension, hypoxaemia,[9] hypercapnia,[10] and epilepsy.[11] In experimental studies, tumour permeability factor[12] and cytokines,[13] prostanoids, polyamines, histamine, bradykinin, serotonin, glutamate, [14-17] and numerous other substances can alter the permeability of the BBB.[18,19] When BBB function is altered, there is an increased diffusion of drugs and other compounds through the BBB. Experimental studies have focused on the role of the membrane P-glycoprotein in cerebral drug elimination, which may have an important action in preventing the accumulation of several drugs in the brain.[20] This hypothesis is supported by the observation that inhibition of the P-glycoprotein seems to increase brain toxicity of several drugs.[21] In the case of BBB alterations, active transport of some drugs, like fentanyl, in and outside the brain tissue, may also be affected.[22] Another mechanism has also been described: BBB disruption secondary to direct tissue injury. This may lead to intracerebral mannitol accumulation if used as a therapeutic intervention.[23] Water conductivity is also increased. This tends to increase the removal of water from diseased tissues by osmotic diuretics.

The relative impermeability of the BBB is one of the mechanisms explaining the effects of osmotic agents: low molecular molecules that do not cross BBB are responsible for the development of osmotic forces across the cerebral capillaries, that can reach an enormous level, thus inducing secondary water movements.

Cerebral protection and resuscitation

Following ischaemic injury, the central nervous system is limited in its regenerative ability. The distinction between protection and resuscitation is made by the time course of the therapeutic intervention.[24,25]

Brain protection has been defined as the "prevention or amelioration of neuronal damage evidenced by abnormalities in cerebral metabolism, histopathology or neurologic function occurring after a hypoxic or an ischaemic event"[26] (that is, treatment that is started before and often sustained throughout the insult).

Brain resuscitation refers to the treatment of the secondary brain injury or simply therapy given after the primary insult. The secondary consequences of ischaemia are those that occur after the cerebral circulation is restored and this period is usually termed "postischaemic injury or reperfusion injury".

As mentioned before, the cellular vulnerability depends on the type of neuron. For example, the limbic system, the pyramidal cells of the CA_1 of the hippocampus, Purkinje cells of the cerebellum, and layers 3, 4, and 6 of the cortex, are extremely vulnerable to ischaemia. Conversely, the cells in the spinal cord seem to resist a longer period of oxygen deprivation without damage.[27]

Research has shown that the intracellular events that occur during ischaemia or after the restoration of circulation and oxygenation contribute to the ultimate neurological damage. Ischaemia produces depolarisation of neurones leading to ionic fluxes (Na^+ and Ca^{2+}) into the cells, probably because of the release of glutamate and aspartate which activates the N-methyl-D-aspartate (NMDA) receptors responsible for the control of the influx of Na^+ and Ca^{2+}. The eventual depletion of all ATP stores leads to failure of the energy-dependent ionic pump system with Na^+ and Ca^{2+} remaining in the cell. The consequences of this intracellular ionic overload result in the formation of prostaglandins, free radicals, mitochondrial respiratory chain paralysis with acidosis, and finally cellular membrane destruction. Ultimately, the goal is to provide effective therapeutic measures that will contribute to the reversal of the cascades of cellular events.

The metabolic requirements of the brain fluctuate and are vitally dependent on continuous CBF for mitochondrial aerobic oxidation of metabolic substrate and membrane stability. The magnitude of the reduced CBF and its duration are the primary determinants of ischaemic injury and subsequent brain failure. Synaptic function will be affected initially as the remaining energy is used to maintain cellular homeostasis and limit interruption of the complex series of biochemical events in the cell. Neuroprotective agents act by either increasing oxygen delivery, reducing oxygen demand or modifying pathological processes such as free radical scavenging, excitatory amino acids (glutamate, aspartate), ionic fluxes, etc., which contribute to secondary brain ischaemia (Table 8.1).

Neuroprotective interactions should ideally be started before the onset of ischaemia. The goal of cerebral protection is to increase the period of time after which irreversible damage will result (Figure 8.2). For example, any cerebral protective regimen that extends the brain's tolerance for anoxia to 10 minutes, would suggest that an ischaemic insult, less than 10 minutes, should be tolerated. However, it is essential for the protective agent to reach the penumbra cells in concentrations large enough to prevent further deterioration, even though the capillary flow is reduced. According to the vulnerability of the neurons involved in the ischaemic process, the therapeutic window for reperfusion of the ischaemic region can be very small (that is 5–15 minutes).[28] It has been shown that if the cerebral tissue is reperfused early, the therapeutic window can be extended up to 12 hours.[29,30] Although studies using the positron emission tomography (PET) scan have suggested that brain cells exposed to very low flow can remain viable up to 48 hours, the prognostic clinical significance of this observation has not been demonstrated.[31]

130

Table 8.1   Methods proposed as protectants against cerebral ischaemia and brain failure.

Metabolism	Capillary flow	Secondary injury	Other
Hypothermia	Hypertension	Glucose control	Thrombolysis
Barbiturates	> Cardiac performance	Hypothermia	Complement cascade
Benzodiazepines		Calcium entry blockers	
	Haemodilution		Vascular bypass
Isoflurane	EDRF	Excitatory amino acids antagonists	
Etomidate	Anticoagulation	Free radical scavengers	
Propofol			
	Rheologic agents	Iron chelation	
Lidocaine	Opioid antagonists	Prostaglandin inhibition	
Opioid agonists			
		Steroids	

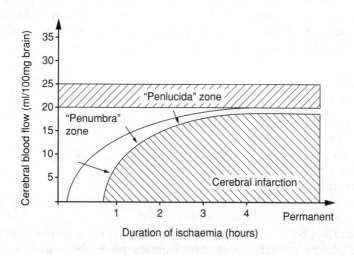

Figure 8.2   Schematic representation of the possible protective effect associated with a therapeutic strategy. The effect of the brain protectants pushes the cerebral infarction zone downward and to the right (black arrows). This suggests that cells in the "penumbra zone" would support reduction in capillary flow for a longer period of time. The time and/or the depth of the critical ischaemic threshold should be modified. However, the earlier the therapy is induced the better the outcome.[32]

Specific treatments in the brain-injured patient

Some of the specific areas of pharmacology used in brain-injured patients are described below.

Hypnotics and sedatives

Indications

The aims of sedation in patients with neurological diseases differ significantly from those in other critically ill patients. In addition to general indications, sedation is a specific part of the medical strategy in the management of brain failure. Treatment aims to provide favourable conditions for the recovery of the damaged brain, while preventing the healthy brain from further secondary brain lesions. To achieve this goal, the choice of sedatives should be limited to drugs that do not interfere with cerebral physiology, particularly the autoregulation of cerebral blood flow, and do not induce unfavourable systemic side effects such as arterial hypotension.

An important aspect of sedation in the patient with neurological involvement is the necessity of a rapid reversal, to allow assessment. The gold standard of neurological monitoring remains the assessment of the level of consciousness and neurological performance. The level of sedation is highly dependent on the clinical condition: deep levels are needed in patients with refractory intracranial hypertension, status epilepticus or suffering from severe acute respiratory failure, while light levels are needed in many non-intubated patients or when a continuous and accurate neurological assessment is mandatory. Undersedation is associated with agitation, intracranial hypertension, stimulation of the sympathetic nervous system, and difficulty in providing intensive care nursing. By contrast, oversedation disturbs neurological assessment and favours arterial hypotension.

Ideal sedative

The ideal sedative[33] is characterised by several properties:

- rapid and smooth onset of action
- rapid reversal
- no effect on cerebral autoregulation and CO_2 reactivity
- decrease in ICP
- decrease in cerebral O_2 consumption
- maintenance of cerebral metabolic/CBF coupling
- absence of significant systemic side effects
- favourable pharmacokinetic properties (small initial distribution volume, high plasma clearance and short elimination half-life, inactive metabolites)
- reasonable cost, taking into account the indirect costs related to drugs with prolonged sedative action, that is, duration of mechanical ventilation and ICU length of stay.

In practice, this ideal drug does not exist. However, some of the commonly used drugs for neurosedation approach this ideal by several of their characteristics. In clinical practice, several classes of hypnotic and sedative drugs are used. Their main effects on the brain and main pharmacokinetic properties are summarised in Tables 8.2 and 8.3.

Hypnotics and sedatives are prescribed to patients with brain failure for four main indications:

- to facilitate mechanical ventilation, induced hypothermia, and other supportive treatments
- to reduce the effects of nociceptive stimuli on ICP and promote ICP control
- to depress cerebral metabolic rate
- to treat epileptic fits.

Benzodiazepines

Benzodiazepines (BDZ) exert their cerebral effect via activation of specific high-affinity binding sites on the γ-aminobutyric acid (GABA)–benzodiazepine receptor complex, which facilitates neurotransmission of GABA. $GABA_\alpha$ receptors show multiple subunits $(\alpha,\beta\gamma,\delta,\rho)$. Special affinity to different classes of sedative depend on this specific subunit affinity and presence. α_4-Subunit expression may be involved in benzodiazepine tolerance and insensitivity.[33,34] Inhibition of the GABA-receptors induces sedation, anxiolysis and amnesia. In addition, benzodiazepines have strong anticomitral effects (see Table 8.2), reduce $CMRO_2$ and CBF by about 30% but have little effect on ICP. They do not abolish cerebral reactivity to CO_2 or autoregulation.[35] The cardiovascular and respiratory effects are usually limited, except in some patients in whom significant arterial hypotension can be induced by even a small IV dose of BDZ.[36] There are great differences in the pharmacokinetics of the various BDZ used in the clinical practice (Tables 8.2 and 8.3). In clinical practice, it is often noticed that the cerebral depressive effect of benzodiazepines and other sedatives is reinforced in patients with brain failure. Furthermore, the elimination half-lives of a given BDZ have a great variability according to the patient and to the clinical circumstances. In clinical practice, midazolam and lorazepam are the most convenient BDZ for intravenous sedation of patients with neurological diseases, because of their short elimination half-lives.[37] However, despite favourable pharmacokinetic properties, the time to recovery after prolonged sedation with these agents is highly variable.[38] Diazepam, a long-acting BDZ, is mainly used for emergency treatment of fits.

Flumazenil is an imidazole benzodiazepine that exerts a competitive action at the benzodiazepine receptor. It antagonises all the effects of BDZ. This property makes flumazenil a useful drug in the diagnosis of benzodiazepine self-poisoning and in the reversal of benzodiazepine over-administration. It has also been shown to partly reverse the effects of hepatic encephalopathy in a small proportion of the patients. However, its relatively short duration of action (half-life 1 to 2 hours) must be kept in

133

Table 8.2 Pharmacokinetic characteristics of some drugs used in the brain injured patient.

Drugs	Vd (L/kg)	$T_{1/2}\beta$ (h)	Clearance (ml/kg/mn)	Protein binding (%)	Metabolism	Route of elimination	Active metabolite
Sedatives and hypnotics							
Midazolam	1·1-2·5	1·5-3·5	4-8	96-98	L	R	No
Lorazepam	1·1	10-20	0·8-1	88-92	L	R	No
Diazepam	0·7-1·7	20-40	0·2-0·5	98	L	R	Yes
Propofol	10	0·5-1	20-30	98	L + Pl	R	No
Ketamine	1·1-2·5	2-4	15-19	47	L	R	Yes
Barbiturates							
Thiopental	1·5-2·5	5-12	3·4-3·6	80	L	R	No
Phenobarbital	0·7	48-96	0·049-0·075	50	L	L and R	Yes
Opiates							
Morphine	3·2	2-4	12-15	35	L	B and R	No
Fentanyl	4	3-4	11-15	79-86	L	B and R	No
Sufentanil	1·7	2-3	13	92	L and G	R	No
Alfentanil	0·9	1-2	2-6	88-92	L	R	No
Remifentanil	0·3-0·4	2	40	70	Pl	R	No
Osmotic agents							
Mannitol	plasma volume	1·5	1·07			R	No
Hypertonic saline			1·07			R	No
Neuroleptics							
Haloperidol	5-10	21	8·9-14·8	92	L	R and E	No
Levomepromazine	30	15-30			L	R and E	No
Calcium antagonists							
Nimodipine	1·3-2·1	0·8-1·4	15-30	99	L	L and E	No
Anticonvulsant agents							
Phenytoin	0·5-0·8	20-40	4·7-7·1	90	L	B and R	No
Clonazepam	2·1-3·3	20-60	1·27-1·83	85	L	B and R	Yes
Other							
Clonidine	1·7-2·5	5-19	1·9-4·3	30-40	L	R and E	No

G = gut; L = liver; R = renal; E = enteral; $T_{1/2}\beta$ = elimination half-life; Vd = distribution volume; B = biliary; Pl = plasma (esterases).

Table 8.3 Practical approach for administration.

Drugs	Route	Initial dose	Subsequent bolus	Infusion rate	Maximum dose per day	Duration	Adjustment RF	Adjustment LF
Hypnotics								
Midazolam	i.v.	0·03–0·2 mg/kg	1–2 mg bolus	0·03–0·2 mg/kg/h		30–60 mn	Yes	Yes
Lorazepam	i.v.	0·02–0·05 mg/kg	1–2 mg bolus		5–6 mg	12–24 h	Yes	No
Diazepam	i.v.	0·1–0·2 mg/kg	2–5 mg bolus		30 mg	12–24 h	Yes	No
Propofol	i.v.	0·3–2 mg/kg	25–50 mg bolus	2·0–10 mg/kg/h	15 mg/kg/h	15–30 mn	No	No
Ketamine	i.v.	0·5–1 mg/kg	25–50 mg bolus	1·0–2·0 mg/kg/h	10 mg/kg	5–15 mn	Yes	Yes
Thiopental	i.v.	3–5 mg/kg	25–50 mg bolus	3·0–10 mg/kg/h		10–20 mn	Yes	Yes
Phenobarbital	p.o.	0·1–0·4 g/d	25–50 mg bolus		0·4 g		Yes	Yes
Opioids								
Morphine	i.v.	0·05–0·1 mg/kg	1–2 mg bolus	0·05–0·15 mg/kg/h		1–2 h	Yes	Yes
Fentanyl	i.v.	0·5–5 mg/kg	25–50 mg bolus	0·5–2 mg/kg/h		30–60 mn	Yes	Yes
Sufentanil	i.v.	0·5–5 mg/kg	10–25 mg bolus			3–5 h	Yes	Yes
Alfentanil	i.v.	10–30 mg/kg	100–250 mg bolus	10–30 mg/kg/h		15–30 mn	No	Yes
Remifentanil	i.v.	1–4 mg/kg	10–25 mg bolus	0·25–2 mg/kg/mn		10–15 mn	No	No
Osmotic agents								
Mannitol	i.v.	0·25–1 g/kg	20 g bolus	2–4 g/h	100–150 g/24 h plasma osmolality	3–8 h	Yes	No
Hypertonic saline	i.v.	100 ml				3–8 h	Yes	No
Neuroleptics								
Haloperidol	i.v.	1–2 mg bolus	1–2 mg bolus		5 mg	3–8 h	No	Yes
Levomepromazine	i.v.	6·25 mg bolus	6·25 mg		50 mg/d	3–8 h	Yes	Yes
Calcium antagonists								
Nimodipine	i.v.	up to 2 mg/h	–	2 mg/h	60 g/d		No	Yes
Anticonvulsant agents								
Phenytoin	i.v.	15 mg/kg	2 mg/kg		1500 mg/d		Yes	Yes
Clonazepam	i.v.	1–2 mg bolus	1–2 mg	0·5 mg/h	4 mg bolus or 20 mg/d	2–3 h	Yes	Yes
Other								
Clonidine	i.v.	1–2·5 µg/kg	1–2·5 µg/kg	0·2–0·5 µg/kg/mn	10–30 µg/kg		Yes	Yes

RF = renal failure; LF = liver failure.

mind, since this may limit its clinical usefulness. The abrupt reversal of BDZ in patients may induce intracranial hypertension in patients with abnormal cerebral compliance[39] and fits in patients after prolonged BDZ administration. Other side effects include anxiety, agitation, and nausea.

Propofol

Propofol is an intravenous sedative with the shortest duration of action and fastest recovery time. Recovery is rapid (15–60 minutes), even after prolonged infusion exceeding 1 week.[40] Its mechanism of action is related to GABA-receptor stimulation. Propofol reduces $CMRO_2$ and CBF, without altering their coupling. Both the cerebral autoregulation and the vascular response to CO_2 stay unaltered during propofol infusion.[41] In patients with increased intracranial pressure, propofol reduces ICP, while preserving CPP, provided arterial hypotension is prevented.[42] Propofol depresses EEG and burst suppression can be obtained. It has strong antiepileptic properties and has been proposed as an alternative to barbiturates in refractory status epilepticus.[43] Based on these properties, propofol may be considered to offer the same degree of cerebral protection as barbiturates during focal ischaemia.[44,45] In the paediatric population, many reports have described propofol toxicity (acidosis, rhabdomyolysis, lung and myocardial injury, convulsions). This contrasts with the adult population, where side effects of propofol are rather uncommon (mostly cardiovascular depression, respiratory failure, acute hyperlipidemia).[46] The latter has been attributed to the excessive lipid load associated with high doses of propofol. The use of propofol 2% solution should decrease lipid load and consequently hyper-lipidemia.

Barbiturates

The main action of barbiturates on CNS function is related to facilitation of GABA transmission. They have cerebral protective properties when given before focal brain ischaemia, but no protective effect in the case of global ischaemia.[47] Among the hypnotics, they produce the greatest reduction of CBF, $CMRO_2$ and ICP in patients with severe brain injury. At high dose, they produce isoelectric EEG, with burst suppression.[48] Because of their prolonged effect and major systemic side effects (arterial hypotension), their administration is limited to severe refractory status epilepticus and refractory intracranial hypertension.[49] In clinical practice, barbiturate dosage is highly variable. Therapy is directed according to the goal. For example, increasing amounts of barbiturates are administered until adequate burst suppression is achieved, in case of brain protection, or until normalisation of ICP, in case of severe head injury.

Opioids

These are often prescribed in combination with short-acting sedatives in patients with neurological injury requiring mechanical ventilation, to limit the cerebral and systemic effects of painful stimuli. Opioids have little effect on cerebral homeostasis, provided $PaCO_2$ changes are prevented by mechanical ventilation.[50]

Neuroleptics

These agents are not widely used owing to their weak sedative effects and their possible side effects, like dyskinesia, and neuroleptic malignant syndrome often confounded with the malignant hyperthermia syndrome. Their use is restricted to patients with acute psychotic syndromes.

Calcium channel antagonists

In addition to the brain injury caused by the initial haemorrhage after a subarachnoid haemorrhage (SAH) the leading causes of morbidity and mortality are arterial vasospasm, rebleeding, and the complications of surgery. The prevention of vasospasm and the reduction of secondary cerebral ischaemia are key points in the therapeutic strategy of SAH.

Numerous pharmacological agents have been shown to exert favourable cerebral effects in experimental models of SAH, reducing the incidence of severe permanent injury due to vasospasm to less than 7%. Pharmacological agents such as calcium blockers, free radical scavengers and corticosteroids, fibrinolytic and/or plasminogen activators, endothelium-relaxing factors, and inhibitors of the complement cascade, have been studied.[51] However, calcium channel antagonists (CCA) are the only agents whose use is supported by controlled studies in patients with SAH. The CCA inhibit calcium transport into cells through the voltage-sensitive ion channel. Some CCA, like nimodipine and nicardipine, act predominantly on cerebral vessels, while many others have effects mainly on systemic vessels.

Nimodipine has been studied in humans with acute stroke, SAH, and after cardiac arrest.[52-54] In SAH, this agent has been shown to decrease both mortality and the incidence of delayed ischaemia and to improve neuro-logical outcome. However, it did not reverse the arterial spasm which per-sisted on angiography. The most favourable effect was observed in patients with moderately severe symptoms, while no effect was observed in cases with severe neurological signs. Favourable outcomes with nimodipine therapy were also reported after stroke. A significant increase in regional CBF in the territory of the ischaemic brain was seen. It was concluded that this perfusion improvement was responsible for an early neurological recovery.

Excitatory amino acid (EAA) antagonists

While the role of EAA and protection by EAA antagonists have been well documented in experimental ischaemia, early clinical studies have been dis-appointing. The prototype non-competitive glutamate antagonist acting at the N-methyl B-aspartate (NMBA) receptor, Dizocilpine (MK-801), never reached large scale clinical trials because of fears about hippocampal neurotoxicity. More recent compounds, either competitive or non-competitive antagonists, have not proved to be effective in outcome trials.

137

Antioxidants

Animal studies have also suggested a prominent role for oxidants in acute brain injury and brain protection by antioxidants. However, studies in humans with pegorgotein and tirilazad have shown no improvement in outcome in clinical head injury.

Hypothermia

Hypothermia decreases the energy requirements of the brain by decreasing both the activation metabolism required for neuronal function, as indicated by electroencephalogram (EEG) activity, and the residual metabolism necessary for the maintenance of cellular integrity. Much interest has focused on mild to moderate hypothermia (33–36°C) as a neuroprotective intervention since animal studies demonstrated improved outcome from cerebral ischaemia.

To date, no large outcome trials have demonstrated benefit from moderate hypothermia. However it is well recognised that an increase in temperature worsens outcome following brain injury and that the prevention of hyperthermia is a highly desirable target in acute brain injury.

Osmotic agents

In the setting of clinical, radiological or measured evidence of intracranial hypertension, mannitol (usually as 20%) 0·25–1·0 gm/kg has traditionally been used to elevate plasma osmolarity and reduce brain oedema. In addition to its use as maintenance fluid, hypertonic saline (7·5%), used for small volume resuscitation, may improve outcome in comatose patients suffering from multiple trauma.[55] Recent reports also highlight the use of 23.4% saline for the treatment of intracranial hypertension.[56]

The mechanisms of action of osmotic agents are complex and not yet completely understood, although several theories have been proposed.

- *Osmotic theory.* This states that hyperosmolar solutions reduce ICP before the loss of interstitial fluid within tissues. The osmotic effectiveness depends on the osmotic reflection coefficient.
- *Haemodynamic theory.* Osmotic agents reduce CBV and hence ICP by decreasing blood viscosity, increasing CPP, or by a combined effect. The resulting reduction of ICP would be maximal if CPP is low and autoregulation preserved. If autoregulation produces constriction of cerebral blood vessels or is severely impaired, limited benefit must be expected from osmotherapy.
- *The diuretic theory.* This believes that the reduction of the plasma volume caused by the osmotic diuresis promotes the jugular venous drainage and induces a parallel reduction of both central venous pressure (CVP) and ICP.

Mannitol may induce cardiovascular side effects: a transient increase in arterial blood pressure, hypervolemia and worsening of congestive heart failure. Systemic dehydration and electrolyte alterations can also complicate mannitol therapy. Because of this, it should be avoided in patients with hyperosmolar states.[57] In patients with compromised renal function, osmotherapy should be used with caution due to the risk of hypervolemia.[58] Some experimental and human studies suggest that mannitol may worsen cerebral hyperemia, consequent to an increase in CBV, although the practical relevance of this phenomenon is difficult to evaluate.[58] There is little rationale in avoiding mannitol in patients with midline shift, since brain water content is decreased in the affected hemisphere as well as in other such circumstances. Since the effects of osmotic agents on disrupted BBB are difficult to predict, rebound swelling is possible, and careful neurological monitoring should be used, including ICP and CT scans when necessary.

Mannitol should be infused through central venous line since it may rapidly induce venous thrombophlebitis. It exerts little effect when ICP is normal. When given to patients with high ICP at doses from 0·25 to 1·5 g/kg (15–30 minutes infusion time), it usually reduces ICP within minutes, although the maximal effect is seen after 20–40 minutes.

Hypertonic saline infusions (3%–7.5%–10%) produce strong osmotic effects. They usually are infused at 100 ml/hour in order to obtain a brain osmotic effect via an increase in plasma osmolality which should not exceed 320 mosmol/l. Hypertonic saline solutions are also used to correct symptomatic hyponatremia. In such conditions, they allow a progressive normalisation of plasma osmolality associated with an expansion of intravascular volume, which must be carefully assessed in order to avoid the development of pulmonary oedema. Hypertonic saline must be avoided in diabetes insipidus and other hyperosmolar states.

Antiepileptic drugs in the management of status epilepticus

Antiepileptic drugs are commonly prescribed in critically ill patients for epileptic seizure control. Status epilepticus (SE) constitutes a life-threatening condition needing prompt management. It is defined as a seizure that persists for a sufficient length of time or is repeated frequently enough that recovery does not occur between attacks.

The goal of medical treatment for SE is the prompt reversal of seizure activity. A recent review has summarised the most important practical aspects of medical management.[58] The main drugs that are currently administered to treat SE include benzodiazepines (midazolam, lorazepam, clonazepam), phenytoin, barbiturates (phenobarbital). In refractory cases, a deep anaesthesia with midazolam, propofol or thiopentone, should be administered.

Midazolam, lorazepam and clonazepam have potent antiepileptic activity and a rapid effect. They are often prescribed as initial treatment of SE, due to their limited systemic side effects.

Phenytoin has not got a rapid effect, due to the time it takes to diffuse across BBB (20–30 minutes to achieve peak brain concentration). It is commonly prescribed for prolonged treatment after seizure reversal by BDZ.

Phenobarbital is not used as a first line drug in SE because of its prolonged depressant effect on CNS and its significant respiratory and cardiovascular effects. Both phenytoin and barbiturates exert a marked induction of the cytochrome P450 system. During prolonged administration, this increases the requirements of many other drugs metabolised via the cytochrome P450 system.

Propofol is the most recent drug released for SE treatment.[48] Its circulatory and metabolic effects on the brain are very similar to those of barbiturates. Its short action is a major advantage, allowing a neurological assessment to be performed shortly after stopping treatment. However, it may have proconvulsant properties. Its definite place in the management of SE is yet unknown. In a recent study performed in epileptic patients undergoing temporal lobe resection, propofol and thiopental administration was associated with equivalent epileptiform activity recorded with electrocorticogram during surgery.[59] These results suggest that propofol has no greater proconvulsive effect than thiopental and constitutes a reasonable alternative treatment for status epilepticus.

Intravenous valproic acid may have a therapeutic effect in patients with refractory epilepsy. Other agents like lidocaine, paraldehyde and chloremethiazole have also been described to terminate status epilepticus. In patients with refractory status epilepticus, several antiepileptic drugs must be combined, like midazolam or propofol, phenytoin and phenobarbital.[59] Such combination carries a high probability of drug interaction, due to the effect on the cytochrome P450 system. The risk can be reduced by frequent monitoring of the drug plasma level.

Special attention must be directed in patients with brain failure to systemic drugs with proconvulsant effects. This is particularly the case for antibiotics like penicillin and carbapenems (thienamycin, meropenem). When administering such agents, it is imperative to avoid rapid injection, which leads to an acute increase in plasma and brain concentrations of these compounds. Attention should be focused on drug level monitoring, particularly in patients with renal or liver failure.

Steroids

Steroids exert potent physiological and pharmacological effects. They are ubiquitous physiological regulators, essential for survival in many stressful situations. The most relevant effects of steroids in patients with neurological injury include: a potent anti-inflammatory action, suppression of immunological response, as well as an effect on intermediate metabolism, fluid and electrolyte balance, and the cardiovascular system. Corticosteroids act on intracellular receptors and many effects are related to post-transcription mechanisms. The cerebral effects are multiple and complex, mainly related to endothelial cell membrane stabilisation, decreased release of toxins and cytokines, facilitation of electrolyte shifts favouring transcapillary movement of fluids, enhanced lysosomal activity of cerebral capillaries, and increased cerebral glucose utilisation, which may improve cerebral function.

In clinical practice, steroids are used to treat cerebral oedema but are not uniformly effective. The therapeutic efficacy of steroids is well demonstrated for perifocal oedema surrounding mass lesions, abscesses, subdural haematoma, bacterial meningitis, and postoperative swelling. They have no proven effect on cerebral oedema associated with brain injury or hypoxic damage and in these conditions, steroids may even worsen the neurological outcome. Steroids decrease CSF formation and facilitate its reabsorption, although the clinical relevance of this effect is yet to be established. This therapeutic action could be used to decrease CBV in cases of high ICP in association with other drugs such as mannitol, diuretics and hyperventilation. The benefits of steroid therapy for cerebral protection in humans remains unproved and controversial.[4] Methylprednisolone and dexamethasone are the most commonly prescribed corticosteroids.

Drugs for cerebral protection

Because of the multifactorial problem involved in cerebral ischaemia, even to date, there are no absolute proven methods of cerebral protection. Brain failure remains the ultimate neurological consequence of an ischaemic insult. The events that take place after the restoration of circulation and reoxygenation must be better understood to optimise the therapy. If these secondary consequences of ischaemia do contribute to the final neurological damage, then therapy must be aimed at preventing these processes. However, to date, there is still little convincing evidence that therapy designed to prevent individual processes is efficacious in limiting cerebral ischaemia and eventually brain failure. Cerebral protection is meant to block these secondary insults, either by prolonging the time of tolerance to ischaemia, or improving capillary flow and oxygenation. Multifactorial therapy such as maintaining adequate cerebral perfusion and oxygen delivery, as well as reducing cellular metabolism, seems largely acceptable to limit the development of brain failure.

Conclusion

Many aspects of brain failure remain unknown, especially when integrity of the BBB is altered. Because the effects of drug administration in this case could lead to unexpected effects, careful monitoring of the patient with brain failure should be performed. This intensive monitoring is based on clinical, electrophysiological, laboratory, and radiological data.

As a baseline routine attitude, the following medical and physiological details are required before administering any drugs to patients with acute neurological disease:

- Identification of the underlying cerebral pathophysiological mechanisms and their local consequences. The most important information concerns the level of consciousness, neurological status, the presence (or risk) of intracranial hypertension, cerebral ischaemia, and convulsion.
- Identification of the associated systemic disturbances which may influence cerebral physiology and drug prescription: arterial hypotension, haemodynamic compromise, abnormal pulmonary gas exchange, water and electrolyte disorders, renal failure, hepatic failure, thermal dysregulation.
- Identification of the expected pharmacological effects of drugs on brain physiology and functions: effects on CBF, $CMRO_2$, $CBF/CMRO_2$ coupling, ICP, autoregulation, reactivity to CO_2, cardiovascular and respiratory effects, effects on conscious level.
- Choice of the appropriate therapeutic strategy: requirement for mechanical ventilation, hypothermia and sedation, intervals for neurological assessment, target for haemodynamic management, temperature regulation, drugs with specific neurological targets.
- Identification of the appropriate systemic therapeutic strategy: treatment of infection, requirement for upper gastrointestinal bleeding prophylactics, artificial nutrition, etc.
- Identification of patients requiring monitoring of drug levels in plasma.

References

1 Werner C, Kochs E, Hoffman WE. Cerebral blood flow and metabolism. In: Albin MS. *Textbook of neuroanesthesia, with neurosurgical and neuroscience perspectives.* New York, London: McGraw-Hill, 1997: 21–59.

2 Benveniste H. The excitotoxin hypothesis in relation to cerebral ischemia. *Cerebrovasc Br Metab Rev* 1991; **3**: 213–45.

3 Lam AM, Winn HR, Cullen BF *et al.* Hyperglycaemia and neurological outcome in patients with head injury. *J Neurosurg* 1991; **75**: 545–51.

4 Artu AA. CSF dynamics, cerebral edema and intracranial pressure. In: Albin MS. *Textbook of neuroanesthesia, with neurosurgical and neuroscience perspectives.* New York, London: McGraw-Hill, 1997: 61–115.

5 Shah GN, Mooradian AD. Age-related changes in the blood–brain barrier. *Exp Gerontol* 1997; **32**: 501–19.

6 Shivers RR, Wijsman JA. Blood–brain barrier permeability during hyperthermia. *Prog Brain Res* 1998; **115**: 413–24.

7 Hartl R, Medary M, Ruge M, Arfors KE, Ghajar J. Blood–brain barrier breakdown occurs early after traumatic brain injury and is not related to white blood cell adherence. *Acta Neurochir Suppl* 1997; **70**: 240–2.

8 Murakami K, Kondo T, Chan PH. Blood–brain barrier disruption, edema formation, and apoptotic neuronal death following cold injury. *Acta Neurochir Suppl* 1997; **70**: 234–6.

9 Strasser A, Stanimirovic D, Kawai N, McCarron RM, Spatz M. Hypoxia modulates free radical formation in brain microvascular endothelium. *Acta Neurochir Suppl* 1997; **70**: 8–11.

10 Mooradian AD, Bastani B. The effect of metabolic acidosis and alkalosis on the H$^+$-ATPase of rat cerebral microvessels. *Life Sci* 1997; **61**: 2247–53.

11 Correale J, Rabinowicz AL, Heck CN, Smith TD, Loskota WJ, DeGiorgio CM. Status epilepticus increases CSF levels of neuron-specific enolase and alters the blood–brain barrier. *Neurology* 1998; **50**: 1388–91.

12 Anda T, Yamashita H, Khalid H *et al.* Effect of tumor necrosis factor-alpha on the permeability of bovine brain microvessel endothelial cell monolayers. *Neurol Res* 1997; **19**: 369–76.

142

13 De Vries HE, Blom-Roosemalen MC, Van Oosten M *et al*. The influence of cytokines on the integrity of the blood–brain barrier *in vitro*. *J Neuroimmunol* 1996; **64**: 37–43.

14 Anthony DC, Bolton SJ, Fearn S, Perry VH. Age-related effects of interleukin-1 beta on polymorphonuclear neutrophil-dependent increases in blood–brain barrier permeability in rats. *Brain* 1997; **120**: 435–44.

15 Easton AS, Fraser PA. Arachidonic acid increases cerebral microvascular permeability by free radicals in single pial microvessels of the anaesthetized rat. *J Physiol* 1998; **507**: 541–7.

16 Glantz L, Nates JL, Trembovler V, Bass R, Shohami E. Polyamines induce blood–brain barrier disruption and edema formation in the rat. *J Basic Clin Physiol Pharmacol* 1996; **7**: 1–10.

17 Mayhan WG, Didion SP. Glutamate-induced disruption of the blood–brain barrier in rats. Role of nitric oxide. *Stroke* 1996; **27**: 965–9.

18 Hurst RD, Clark JB. Nitric oxide-induced blood–brain barrier dysfunction is not mediated by inhibition of mitochondrial respiratory chain activity and/or energy depletion. *Nitric Oxide* 1997; **1**: 121–9.

19 Hurst RD, Clark JB. Alterations in transendothelial electrical resistance by vasoactive agonists and cyclic AMP in a blood–brain barrier model system. *Neurochem Res* 1998; **23**: 149–54.

20 Jonker JW, Wagenaar E, Van Deemter L *et al*. Role of blood–brain barrier P-glycoprotein in limiting brain accumulation and sedative side-effects of asimadoline, a peripherally acting analgesic drug. *Br J Pharmacol* 1999; **127**: 43–50.

21 Fenart L, Buee-Scherrer V, Descamps L *et al*. Inhibition of P-glycoprotein: rapid assessment of its implication in blood–brain barrier integrity and drug transport to the brain by an *in vitro* model of the blood–brain barrier. *Pharm Res* 1998; **15**: 993–1000.

22 Henthorn TK, Liu Y, Mahapatro M, Ng KY. Active transport of fentanyl by the blood–brain barrier. *J Pharmacol Exp Ther* 1999, **289**: 1084–9.

23 McManus ML, Soriano SG. Rebound swelling of astroglial cells exposed to hypertonic mannitol. *Anesthesiology* 1998; **88**: 1586–91.

24 Schell R. Cerebral protection and neuroanesthesia. In: Bissonnette B, ed. *Cerebral protection, resuscitation and monitoring: a look into the future of neuroanesthesia. Anesthesiology Clinics of North America*. Philadelphia: WB Saunders, 1992: 453–70.

25 Milde Newberg L. Cerebral resuscitation, is it possible? In: Bissonnette B, ed. *Cerebral protection, resuscitation and monitoring: a look into the future of neuroanesthesia. Anesthesiology Clinics of North America*. Philadelphia: WB Saunders, 1992: 575–603.

26 Messick JM, Milde LN. Brain protection. *Adv Anesthesia* 1987; **4**: 47–61.

27 Hossmann KA. Post-ischemic resuscitation of the brain: selective vulnerability versus global resistance. *Prog Brain Res* 1985; **63**: 3–17.

28 Pulsinelli, WA. The therapeutic window in ischemic brain injury. *Curr Op Neurol* 1995; **8**: 3–5.

29 Heiss WD. Experimental evidence of ischemic thresholds and functional recovery. *Stroke* 1992; **23**: 1668–72.

30 Heiss WD, Fink GR, Huber M, Herholz K. Positron emission tomography imaging and the therapeutic window. *Stroke* 1993; **24**: 50–3.

31 Heiss WD, Graf R. The ischemic penumbra. *Curr Op Neurol* 1994; **7**: 11–19.

32 Bissonnette B. Cerebral protection in children. *Paediatr Anaesth*, 1997.

33 Hevers W, Luddens H. The diversity of GABAA receptors. Pharmacological and electrophysiological properties of GABAA channel subtypes. *Mol Neurobiol* 1998; **18**: 35–86.

34 Luddens H, Korpi ER. Biological function of GABAA/benzodiazepine receptor heterogeneity. *J Psychiatr Res* 1995; **29**: 77–94.

35 Strebel S, Kaufmann M, Guardiola PM, Schaefer HG. Cerebral vasomotor responsiveness to carbon dioxide is preserved during propofol and midazolam anesthesia in humans. *Anesth Analg* 1994; **78**: 884–8.

36 Papazian L. Albanese J, Thirion X, Perrin G, Durbec O, Martin C. Effect of bolus doses of midazolam on intracranial pressure and cerebral perfusion pressure in patients with severe head injury. *Br J Anaesth* 1993; **71**: 267–71.

37 Pohlman AS, Simpsdon KP, Hall JB. Continuous intravenous infusions of lorazepam versus midazolam for sedation during mechanical ventilatory support: a prospective, randomized study. *Crit Care Med* 1994; **22**: 1241–7.

38 Backman JT, Olkkola KT, Aranko K, Himberg JJ, Neuvonen PJ. Dose of midazolam should be reduced during kiltiazem and verapamil treatments. *Br J Clin Pharmacol* 1994; **37**: 221–5.

39 Chiolero RL, De Tribolet N. Sedatives and antagonists in the management of severely head-injured patients. *Acta Neurochir Suppl* 1992; **55**: 43–6.

40 Beller JP, Pottecher T, Lugnier A, Mangin P, Otteni JC. Prolonged sedation with propofol in ICU patients: recovery and blood concentration changes during periodic interruptions in infusion. *Br J Anaesth* 1988; **61**: 583–8.

41 Lagerkranser M, Stange K, Sollevi A. Effects of propofol on cerebral blood flow, metabolism, and cerebral autoregulation in the anesthetized pig. *J Neurosurg Anesthesiol* 1997; **9**: 188–93.

42 Nimkoff L, Quinn C, Silver P, Sagy M. The effects of intravenous anesthetics on intracranial pressure and cerebral perfusion pressure in two feline models of brain edema. *J Crit Care* 1997; **12**: 132–6.

43 Wang B, Bai Q, Jiao X, Wang E, White PF. Effect of sedative and hypnotic doses of propofol on the EEG activity of patients with or without a history of seizure disorders. *J Neurosurg Anesthesiol* 1997; **9**: 335–40.

44 Young Y, Menon DK, Tisavipat N, Matta BF, Jones JG. Propofol neuroprotection in a rat model of ischaemia reperfusion injury. *Eur J Anaesthesiol* 1997; **14**: 320–6.

45 Zhu H, Cottrell JE, Kass IS. The effect of thiopental and propofol on NMDA- and AMPA-mediated glutamate excitotoxicity. *Anesthesiology* 1997; **87**: 944–51.

46 Miller LJ, Wiles-Pfeifler R. Propofol for the long-term sedation of a critically ill patient. *Am J Crit Care* 1998; **7**: 73–6.

47 Amakawa K, Adachi N, Liu K, Ikemune K, Fujitani T, Arai T. Effects of pre- and postischemic administration of thiopental on transmitter amino acid release and histologic outcome in gerbils. *Anesthesiology* 1996; **85**: 1422–30.

48 Akrawi WP, Drummond JC, Kalkman CJ, Patel PM. A comparison of the electrophysiologic characteristics of EEG burst-suppression as produced by isoflurane, thiopental, etomidate, and propofol. *J Neurosurg Anesthesiol* 1996; **8**: 40–6.

49 Steen PA. Barbiturates in neuroanesthesia and neuro-intensive care. *Agressologie* 1991; **32**: 323–5.

50 Herrick IA, Gelb AW, Manninen PH, Reichman H, Lownie S. Effects of fentanyl, sufentanil, and alfentanil on brain retractor pressure. *Anesth Analg* 1991; **72**: 359–63.

51 Feigin VL, Rinkel GJ, Algra A, Vermeulen M, Van Gijn J. Calcium antagonists in patients with aneurysmal subarachnoid hemorrhage: a systematic review. *Neurol* 1998; **50**: 876–83.

52 Gelmers HJ, Hennerici M. Effect of nimodipine on acute ischemic stroke. Pooled results from five randomized trials. *Stroke* 1990; **21**(suppl): IV81–4.

53 Robinson MJ, Teasdale GM. Calcium antagonists in the management of subarachnoid haemorrhage. *Cerebrovasc Br Metab Rev* 1990; **2**: 205–26.

54 Roine RO, Kaste M, Kinnunen A, Nikki P, Sarna S, Kajaste S. Nimodipine after resuscitation from out-of-hospital ventricular fibrillation. A placebo-controlled, doubleblind, randomized trial. *JAMA* 1990; **264**: 3171–7.

55 Vasser MJ, Fischer RP, O'Brien PE *et al*. A multicentre trial for resuscitation of head injured patients with 7·5% sodium chloride. The effect of added dextram 70. The Multicenter Group for the Study of Hypertonic Saline in Trauma Patients. *Arch Surg* 1993; **128**: 1003–11.

56 Suarez JI, Qureshi AI, Bhardwaj A *et al*. Treatment of refractory intracranial hypertension with 23·4% saline. *Crit Care Med* 1998; **26**: 1118–22.

57 Kaufmann AM, Cardoso ER. Aggravation of vasogenic cerebral edema by multiple-dose mannitol. *J Neurosurg* 1992; **77**: 584–9.

58 Lowenstein DH, Alldredge BK. Status epilepticus. *N Engl J Med* 1998; **338**: 970–6.

59 Hewitt PB, Chu DLK, Polkey CE, Binnie CD. Effects of propofol on the electrocorticogram in epileptic patients undergoing cortical resection. *Br J Anaesth* 1999; **82**: 199–202.

9: Respiratory failure

MAIRE SHELLY

Introduction

Acute respiratory failure is a major factor precipitating admission to an intensive care unit (ICU) and chronic pulmonary disease is a common comorbidity in critically ill patients. Alterations in the pharmacokinetics of drugs can arise because of the pulmonary disease itself and because of associated factors such as hypoxia and mechanical ventilation. Other associated factors may also contribute, for example, cigarette smoking induces certain enzymes and can in itself alter drug metabolism.[1] This chapter reviews the pharmacokinetic consequences of respiratory disease and its treatment.

Respiratory disease

Respiratory disease can alter pharmacokinetics in a number of factors, including:

- hypoxia
- hypercapnia
- acid–base problems
- right ventricular dysfunction
- altered regional blood flow
- pulmonary alveolar dysfunction.

Often, a combination of these factors will affect the absorption, distribution, and elimination of drugs.

Absorption

Regional blood flow is altered in respiratory disease for several reasons. Hypoxaemia will lead to increased blood flow to essential organs whilst tachypnoea and dyspnoea will increase blood flow to the respiratory muscles. These changes will divert blood flow from areas of drug absorption, such as the gastrointestinal tract (GIT), rectum, and gluteal muscles, and will, in turn, reduce drug absorption. Alterations in splanchnic blood flow can reduce absorption of orally administered bronchodilators. A decreased absorption of theophylline, salbutamol, and terbutaline has been reported in patients with respiratory disease after oral administration.[2-6] This is manifest as reduced plasma concentrations at night when patients are most at risk. There is also an increase in trough concentration in the morning as blood flow to the GIT is stimulated by breakfast with the potential for drug toxicity. A decrease in gastric emptying and sleeping in the supine position may contribute to the decreased absorption.

The oral bioavailability of salbutamol and terbutaline is normally low since there is extensive metabolism of both drugs in the gut wall.[7] Both drugs have enantiomers and this metabolic process is stereospecific.[8] These drugs are normally given by other routes to avoid any further reduction in absorption as a result of reduced splanchnic blood flow. When splanchnic perfusion is reduced, there is an associated reduction in the metabolic processes of the liver or GIT.[9] Any drug with significant first-pass metabolism may have an increased bioavailability.

Inhaled drugs

When drugs are administered by the inhaled route, it is necessary for an adequate amount of drug to reach its site of action, usually the small airways. The amount of drug reaching this site is usually about 15% of the inhaled dose; the remainder is deposited in large airways and has no clinical effect.[10] Factors that influence the distribution of inhaled particles within the lung are:

- *Particle size.* Smaller particles reach further down the airways, larger particles are deposited in the large airways.
- *Speed of inhalation.* A rapid flow into the airways will tend to wash particles further down the large airways where gas flow is laminar. This relationship is less applicable when gas flow becomes turbulent since particles may then have more contact with the airway wall.
- *Tidal volume.* A greater proportion of inhaled particles will reach the alveoli with a large tidal volume since alveolar ventilation is greater and dead space ventilation proportionally reduced.
- *Duration of the inspiratory pause.* During the inspiratory pause, alveoli are recruited for gas exchange. Alveolar ventilation is enhanced and inhaled particles are more likely to reach the lower airways.

Patients with respiratory disease have altered respiratory dynamics and often have a poor inhalation technique. One result of this is that more of any inhaled agent will be deposited in the large airways and be clinically ineffective.[11,12] An example is sodium chromoglycate. This drug has minimal absorption from the GIT and inhaled administration is essential. Absorption from the lungs is related to inspiratory flow rate and can be increased by manoeuvres to improve lung function.[13] Absorption of inhaled salbutamol is increased in patients with cystic fibrosis. The reason for this is unclear but may be related to a higher permeability of the chronically inflamed small and large airways.[14]

Pentamidine is used in the management of *Pneumocystis carinii* pneumonia, particularly in patients with acquired immunodeficiency syndrome

146

(AIDS). It is poorly absorbed from the GIT and after intravenous infusion, pharmacokinetics suggest a high tissue uptake[15] confirmed by high tissue concentrations.[16] Aerosol administration produces higher concentrations in bronchoalveolar fluid and these concentrations are maintained for longer.[17] There is wide variation between individuals, and patients undergoing mechanical ventilation have higher plasma concentrations after an aerosol dose than do spontaneously breathing subjects.[18] This may be because of reduced drug loss in the breathing system, more effective nebulisation with smaller particle sizes, or increased uptake through the alveolar capillary membrane owing to pulmonary disease.

Distribution

The process by which drugs reach their site of action may be altered in patients with respiratory disease for several reasons.

The volume of distribution of a drug varies with its degree of protein binding, since only free drug is able to cross membranes. The proteins predominantly concerned with drug carriage are albumin and α_1-acid glycoprotein, the concentrations of both vary with respiratory disease. α_1-acid glycoprotein is an acute phase protein and its concentration increases in many inflammatory and infective processes within the lung, specifically chronic obstructive pulmonary disease (COPD), inflammatory lung diseases, lung cancer, and respiratory infections.[19] Propranolol is carried on α_1-acid glycoprotein and unbound propranolol concentrations in elderly patients with respiratory disease are half that of normal volunteers. This is attributed to increased α_1-acid glycoprotein concentrations.[20]

Albumin is also important in drug carriage and its concentration is reduced in critically ill patients. Theophylline binding is linearly related to albumin concentration and is reduced in critically ill patients compared with patients with COPD.[21]

Drugs with a pK_a close to the value of plasma pH have a degree of ionisation sensitive to small changes in plasma pH. This will also change their volume of distribution. Theophylline protein binding is sensitive to pH; 30% is bound at a plasma pH of 7·0 and 65% at a pH of 7·8.[22]

Drugs given parenterally or orally need effective distribution to reach their site of action in the lung. Antibiotics, in particular, need effective penetration from plasma to sputum.[23] This will be affected by the physicochemical properties of drug, such as pK_a and lipid solubility, as well as the diffusion gradient for the drug, which will depend on the plasma concentration. Another factor is the integrity of the bronchial mucosa and alveolar membrane. Penetration of these membranes may be increased in inflammatory lung diseases.[24] This has been reported for some antibiotics, including, ampicillin, amoxycillin, cephalexin and tobramycin but not for others such as gentamicin. It has been suggested that the sputum concentration of an antibiotic may be a more relevant measure of effectiveness than serum concentration, which is a better measure of toxicity.[25]

Patients with cystic fibrosis have altered pharmacokinetics of antibiotics.

147

There is a decreased maximum plasma concentration, a decreased area under the plasma concentration–time curve, and a shorter elimination half-life than normal. These changes are caused by an increased volume of distribution and changes in metabolism and elimination.[26]

Elimination

The major routes of drug elimination are the liver and kidney. However, the importance of other routes of elimination, such as the GIT and the lung itself, is now being realised. There is enormous variability in the rate of drug clearance in normal subjects. In patients with respiratory disease, this variability is increased. For example, the variability in theophylline clearance is increased during an acute respiratory illness in both adults and children.[27,28]

Hepatic drug clearance depends on liver blood flow, the intrinsic metabolic capacity of the liver and the degree of protein binding. Liver blood flow may be reduced as a result of reduced splanchnic blood flow or reduced cardiac output. Cardiac output can be reduced secondary to right ventricular failure in severe lung pathology or during mechanical ventilation. This is discussed later. The metabolic capacity of the liver is unchanged in uncomplicated asthma or COPD and there are no clinically important problems with drug metabolism.[29] Problems with metabolic capacity are often associated with hypoxia (discussed later). Protein-binding changes are as described in the section on distribution. A greater free-drug fraction will result in some increase in clearance but the extent of this increase will depend on the extraction ratio of the drug (see Chapter 2).

Renal elimination of drugs in patients with pulmonary disease has not been studied. In theory, the main factors which decrease renal elimination are a decreased cardiac output and renal blood flow secondary to either right heart failure or mechanical ventilation or a reduced renal extraction.[30] A reduced renal blood flow will reduce clearance of drugs that depend on glomerular filtration for their clearance. Examples include vancomycin, aminoglycosides, and digoxin; toxicity may develop for all three if plasma concentrations are not closely monitored. Drugs that depend on tubular secretion for their elimination also need an adequate renal blood flow so that tubular perfusion is maintained. If renal blood flow decreases, their elimination will also decrease. A further circumstance occurs with drugs that are reabsorbed in the renal tubules, for instance, aminoglycosides. In patients with oliguria, the drug concentration in the urine increases and this in turn increases the gradient for drug reabsorption and less drug is eliminated.

The lungs are involved in the elimination of many drugs and endogenous substances and are important because they receive the whole cardiac output. Within the lungs, different cell populations appear to be responsible for different metabolic pathways. Pulmonary clearance is influenced by a number of factors.[31] Cigarette smoking induces several enzyme systems and can enhance clearance; for example, theophylline clearance is increased in smokers.[32] Pulmonary clearance also varies with changes in cardiac output and ventilation/perfusion abnormalities. Plasma pH changes may alter the ability of the lung to clear circulating substances; for example, the pulmonary clearance of mescaline is increased in respiratory alkalosis. Another factor is the integrity of the pulmonary capillary cell. In acute lung injury there is a decreased removal of endogenous alprostadil and serotonin.[33,34]

Ventilation

During positive pressure ventilatory support, intrathoracic pressure becomes positive rather than negative and this has a number of physiological consequences[30] as follows:

- decreased cardiac output
    decreased stroke volume
    decreased ventricular filling
    increased pulmonary vascular resistance
    decreased myocardial contractility
- decreased hepatic blood flow
- decreased splanchnic blood flow
- decreased renal blood flow
    decreased glomerular filtration
    decreased sodium excretion
    decreased free water clearance
    decreased urine output.

Because different modes of ventilation have different effects on intrathoracic pressure, the overall effect of ventilation on drug pharmacokinetics will depend on several factors.

- *Ventilation mode.* Generally the higher the intrathoracic pressure, the more pronounced the physiological consequences. Aggressive positive pressure ventilation will therefore have more profound effects on pharmacokinetics than ventilatory modes with pressure limitations.
- *Pulmonary pathology.* A decrease in lung compliance caused by the respiratory disease process will lead to a greater increase in intrathoracic pressure than usual if the patient requires ventilatory support. This will in turn cause greater physiological and pharmacokinetic disturbances.
- *Drug used.* The pharmacokinetics of different drugs will differ in their sensitivity to the physiological changes produced by mechanical ventilation.
- *Haemodynamic status.* Effective resuscitation manoeuvres, such as expansion of the intravascular volume or inotropic support, will maintain haemodynamic stability. This in turn will minimise the physiological and pharmacokinetic consequences of mechanical ventilation.

As the patient's condition improves and ventilatory support is weaned, pharmacokinetic changes may occur with pharmacodynamic consequences.

149

Absorption

Since mechanical ventilation reduces splanchnic blood flow, there may be decreased absorption of drugs given orally. The amount of drug entering the systemic circulation may be maintained in spite of a decreased absorption because of a decrease in first-pass metabolism. These changes are similar to those seen with respiratory disease. If a patient's lungs are being ventilated for respiratory disease, changes in absorption may be more profound.

Distribution

During ventilation, there is an increase in total body water. This is caused by a reduced glomerular filtration and urine output secondary to a decreased renal blood flow as well as salt and water retention secondary to release of antidiuretic hormone and atrial natriuretic factor. The increased body water leads to a higher volume of distribution of more water-soluble drugs. For example, patients had a higher volume of distribution of gentamicin while undergoing controlled ventilation after cardiopulmonary bypass than they did after weaning from ventilatory support. The volume of distribution of gentamicin was also higher in the group of patients whose ventilation was supported than in a control group who were breathing spontaneously throughout.[35] An increased volume of distribution of drugs such as gentamicin may result in the peak plasma concentrations being subtherapeutic.

Elimination

Mechanical ventilation by itself has no effect on the intrinsic metabolic capacity of an organ; in fact, by improving oxygenation, it may increase metabolic capacity (see later). Protein binding is also unaffected, although many patients needing ventilatory support will have altered protein concentrations. The main effect of mechanical ventilation on drug clearance is as a result of altered regional perfusion. Therefore, the drugs most likely to be affected are those whose clearance is dependent on hepatic blood flow.

There are few studies on the effects of ventilation on drug clearance. The clearance of lignocaine is decreased by 22% in patients whose lungs were mechanically ventilated compared with its clearance in the same patients after weaning.[36] This is associated with an increase of 35% in the half-life and of 24% in the serum concentration of lignocaine. There may be changes to a similar extent in other drugs with a high extraction ratio, for instance, labetolol, pethidine, and verapamil.

The decreased renal blood flow during ventilation is important in the clearance of drugs predominantly eliminated by glomerular filtration such as vancomycin, digoxin, and aminoglycosides. Amikacin clearance has been shown to be proportional to glomerular filtration rate[37] and tobramycin clearance was increased by 20% when renal perfusion was increased using a dopamine infusion.[38]

150

Drugs such as digoxin and frusemide, which undergo tubular secretion, will also be affected by changes in renal blood flow because of secondary changes in tubular blood flow.[39] As well as that, drugs that undergo tubular reabsorption, such as aminoglycosides and theophylline, will have increased reabsorption as the urine output decreases and concentration of the drug in the urine increases.[40,41]

Hypoxaemia

Oxygen is vital for cellular metabolism and is a substrate for many reactions. These are particularly oxygenase reactions involving cytochrome P450 enzymes and oxidase reactions where oxygen is an electron acceptor (see Chapter 2). Many processes also depend on the state of oxidation of the cell, the redox state. Hypoxia will, therefore, have profound effects on drug clearance but may also influence absorption and distribution. Respiratory problems can lead to both simple hypoxia where organ blood flow is maintained or stagnant hypoxia where organ blood flow is altered in addition.

Absorption

Drug absorption from the gastrointestinal tract may be reduced in hypoxia. A reduction in oxygen delivery to the GIT may lead to decreased GIT motility or to atrophy of the absorptive villous mucosa lining the GIT. As a result, drug absorption will decrease. Hypoxia, for example, leads to a decreased absorption of paracetamol from the gastrointestinal tract.[42,43] The reduced absorption of an orally administered drug may be partly compensated for by reduced first-pass metabolism secondary to hepatic hypoxia (see below). This may maintain drug bioavailability.

Distribution

Distribution of drugs in the hypoxaemic patient may also be altered. Reduced oxygen delivery to vital organs results in changes in regional blood flow and alterations in body water distribution. Both these factors alter the volume of distribution of a drug. The kidneys are particularly at risk of hypoxic damage and impaired renal function leads to an increased volume of distribution of hydrophilic drugs because of water and sodium retention.

Elimination

Some of the most important changes that occur as a result of hypoxia are those in drug metabolism and elimination. The metabolism of drugs with a low extraction ratio depends on the metabolic capacity of the metabolising organ. Hypoxia predominantly affects metabolic capacity although changes in organ blood flow are important and have already been mentioned.

The liver has an acinar structure based around a vascular axis with peripheral venous drainage. Acinar perfusion is unidirectional so there are gradients of oxygen, glucose, metabolites, and hormones from the centre to the periphery. The acinus is arbitrarily divided into three zones (Figure 9.1):

151

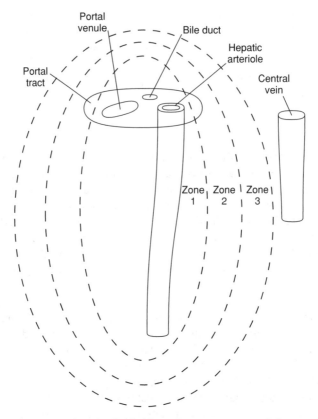

Figure 9.1   The liver acinus is divided into three zones around the arterial supply. Zone 1 is adjacent to the artery and has the best oxygen supply. Zones 2 and 3 are peripheral to zone 1 and are more hypoxic, even under normal conditions. Gradients of substrates and enzymes also occur across the zones.

zone 1 adjacent to the central vascular supply, zone 2 peripheral to this, and zone 3 the most peripheral. As well as the gradients of substrates, there are gradients of enzymes and receptors across the zones. For example, sulphation occurs predominantly in zone 1 whereas the total activity of cytochrome P450 enzymes increases from zone 1 to zone 3.[44] Under hypoxic conditions, the gradient of oxygen from zone 1 to zone 3 becomes steeper with zones 2 and 3 being increasingly sensitive to hypoxia.[45]

The cytochrome P450 enzyme system is normally saturated with oxygen; however, oxidases and oxygenases have a differing dependence on oxygen[46] and their function will be altered differently by differing degrees of hypoxia. This may reflect the distribution of enzymes within the acinus and different oxygen concentrations in their normal environment. A substrate binding to a P450 enzyme alters the spin state of the haem iron from the ferric to the ferrous form. The ferric form is regenerated by binding oxygen to oxidise and then releases the drug.[45] Since both oxygen and substrate share a binding site, the nature of the substrate will also affect the affinity of the enzyme for oxygen and render the reaction sensitive to even mild hypoxia. Where enzyme reactions are directly sensitive to hypoxia, the term metabolic hypoxia is used.[47]

Conjugation reactions are not directly dependent on oxygen but may be affected by hypoxia nevertheless. Hypoxia decreases the function of cytochrome oxidase, which in turn decreases the available energy in the cell and decreases the rate of energy-dependent drug metabolism.[47] Conjugation reactions require energy in the form of ATP and so are affected by hypoxia. This is termed bioenergetic hypoxia and these reactions are generally less sensitive to hypoxia than reactions where metabolic hypoxia is important.[47]

Reactions with a low affinity for oxygen are affected by hypoxia before those with a higher affinity.[46] Thus methylation and sulphation are more vulnerable to hypoxia than glucuronidation, acetylation, and glutathione conjugation. The selectivity of response to bioenergetic hypoxia depends on the relative affinity of the system for ATP. Again, those with the greatest affinity are relatively spared as hypoxia develops.

In bioenergetic hypoxia, available NAD^+, $NADPH$, $NADH$, and $NADP^+$ are also reduced. These are cofactors for many reactions including glucuronidation reactions. Maintenance of intracellular cofactor balance is dependent on energy and thus oxygen. The ratios of oxidative and reductive cofactors are altered in hypoxia and the metabolic processes involving these cofactors are decreased.[47] Intracellular oxygen gradients may develop under hypoxic conditions and lead to differing degrees of reduced activity in different enzyme groups.[48] A situation where hypoxia has a different effect is erythropoietin production. Erythropoietin is responsible for red cell production and hypoxia is an important stimulus for its release. The gene for erythropoietin production has an oxygen-sensing system at the level of transcription. This stimulates production of erythropoietin in response to prolonged hypoxia rather than acute hypoxia. A similar system has been found in other mammalian cells which may mediate other responses to hypoxia at the transcription level.[43] For instance, during the stress response, acute phase proteins are produced and there is reduced production of other proteins such as some cytochrome P450 enzymes. Since hypoxia and stress are linked, production of stress proteins may be initiated in a manner similar to that of erythropoietin.

The metabolism of certain drugs is increased in hypoxia. Misonidazole is a member of the imidazole group of antifungal agents and is used as a radiation-sensitising agent that binds to hypoxic cells. The clearance of misonidazole increases three- to fourfold in hypoxia and different metabolites are produced. Hypoxic conditions lead to reductive metabolic pathways being potentiated to such an extent that they greatly exceed the oxidative metabolism of misonidazole.[49] A similar situation has been reported with omeprazole. Production of the oxidative sulphone metabolite decreased in parallel with the clearance of the parent drug as the oxygen supply was progressively decreased. Production of the reductive sulphide metabolite, however, increased linearly with increasing hypoxia.[50] It is also suggested that reductive metabolites may have an increased ability to damage cellular mechanisms.[45]

Whilst the metabolism of many drugs, such as midazolam, decreases with hypoxia,[51] for others there may be some adaptation to hypoxic conditions with time. Animals rendered acutely hypoxic have reduced clearance of hexobarbitone and pentobarbitone. However, if the animals are exposed to normoxia after five days of hypoxia, clearance of hexobarbitone and pento-barbitone is increased in comparison with animals maintained in normoxia throughout.[47,52–56] Chronic hypoxia also decreased the glucuronidation and sulphation of paracetamol to 60–70% of normal, whereas oxygen therapy increased the concentration of metabolites.[57] Conjugation with glutathione was unchanged from control values and this could contribute to toxicity, particularly if glutathione levels are reduced by hypoxia in man as they are in the rat.[58] The apparent reversibility of some reactions with hypoxia may be because the enzyme is rendered inactive rather than destroyed.[58] These studies also suggest that hypoxia can induce at least some drug metabolis-ing systems[59,60] and this may account for some of the differences in the response to acute and chronic hypoxia.

Toxicity may result from oxygen dependence for different reasons.[61] There may be an increase in toxicity as oxygen concentration is increased. This is usually because of production of a toxic metabolite, for example, the production of p-benzoquinoneimine from paracetamol, or the produc-tion of free radicals. Other metabolic products are more toxic under hypoxic conditions. For example, halogenated hydrocarbon inhalational anaesthetic agents are more toxic under hypoxic conditions than under normoxia or anoxia. This is the result of a reductive metabolic step that requires oxygen and is potentiated by hypoxia. Electron transfer to the halogenated hydrocarbon causes release of a halide ion and generates a free radical that initiates cell damage. In the case of midazolam, metabo-lism is decreased with hypoxia[51] and is virtually absent with anoxia.[62] Metabolism of midazolam is also decreased with a combination of hyper-oxia and propofol.[62] The presence of oxygen allows the free radical pro-duction to be amplified so maximal tissue injury occurs with hypoxia rather than anoxia. Hyperoxia, however, may lead to other metabolic pathways so the first metabolic step does not occur and toxicity is avoided.[61] Toxicity may also be produced if hypoxic cells have an enhanced susceptibility to oxidant injury as a result of suppressed homeo-static functions.[61]

Renal metabolism is affected by hypoxia in an analogous manner. Oxygen gradients within the kidney are significant.[63] Renal tissue oxygen levels are considerably less than renal arterial levels, possibly because of intrarenal shunts and areas of the kidney are at significant risk of hypoxia, even under normal circumstances.[64] The kidney has a variety of enzyme systems that are sensitive to metabolic and bioenergetic hypoxia but these systems have not been investigated.

Other factors

Other factors in the physiology or treatment of respiratory disease may have an effect on the pharmacokinetics of drugs. These factors have not been studied but some effect may be predicted.

Management of acute respiratory distress syndrome often includes ventilation with nitric oxide and nursing the patient in a prone position to improve oxygenation. Both these factors will alter the ventilation/perfusion matching within the lung and therefore could alter absorption of inhaled agents. Improvements in oxygenation may increase clearance and any reduction in ventilatory pressures may improve splanchnic blood flow. Significant changes in pharmacokinetics could result. The medical treatment of respiratory disease is growing rapidly and many patients receive more than one agent for their illness. The interactions of different drugs is outside the remit of this chapter but may cause problems.

Conclusion

Patients with chronic pulmonary disease often have little pharmacokinetic abnormality as a result. This may be because of adaptations, particularly in drug clearance over time. However, patients with an acute respiratory problem may have significantly altered pharmacokinetics of drugs given to treat their illness. This is particularly the case if the patient requires mechanical ventilation or is hypoxic. In this situation it is often difficult to separate the respiratory problem from other organ dysfunction as a result of hypoxia. The effects of respiratory disease on drug pharmacokinetics are variable and different patients behave in very different ways. It is therefore essential to monitor the effect of any drug given and, if toxicity is a risk, to obtain plasma concentrations.

1 Miller L. Recent developments in the study of the effects of cigarette smoking on clinical pharmacokinetics and clinical pharmacodynamics. *Clin Pharmacokinet* 1989;**17**:90–108.
2 Warren JB, Cuss F, Barnes PJ. Posture and theophylline kinetics. *Br J Clin Pharmacol* 1985;**19**:707–9.
3 Jackson SHD, Johnston A, Woollard R, Abrams SML, Turner P. Circadian variation in theophylline absorption during chronic dosing with slow release theophylline preparation and the effect of clock time dosing. *Br J Clin Pharmacol* 1988;**26**:73–7.
4 Jonkman JHG, Borgstrom L, Van der Boon WJV, De Noord OE. Theophylline–terbutaline, a steady state study on possible pharmacokinetic interactions with special reference to chronopharmacokinetic aspects. *Br J Clin Pharmacol* 1988;**26**:285–93.
5 Powell ML, Weisberger M, Dowdy Y *et al.* Comparative steady state bioavailability of conventional and controlled-release formulations of albuterol. *Biopharm Drug Dispos* 1987;**8**:461–8.
6 Pauwels R, Elinck W, Lamont H, Van der Straeten M, Ljungholm K. A comparison of the clinical and bronchodilating effects of plain and slow-release tablets of terbutaline at steady state. *Br J Clin Pharmacol* 1986;**21**:217–22.
7 George CF. Drug metabolism by the gastro-intestinal mucosa. *Clin Pharmacokinet* 1981;**6**:259–74.
8 Borgstrom L, Nyberg L, Jonsson S, Lindberg C, Paulson J. Pharmacokinetic evaluation in man of terbutaline given as separate enantiomers and as the racemate. *Br J Clin Pharmacol* 1989;**27**:49–56.

9 Taburet A-M, Tollier C, Richard C. The effect of respiratory disorders on clinical pharmacokinetic variables. *Clin Pharmacokinet* 1990;**19**:462–90.

10 Clay MM, Clarke SW. Wastage of drug from nebulisers: a review. *J R Soc Med* 1987;**80**:38–9.

11 Brain JD, Valberg PA. Disposition of aerosol in the respiratory tract. *Am Rev Respir Dis* 1979;**120**:1325–73.

12 Newman SP. Aerosol deposition considerations in inhalation therapy. *Chest* 1985;**88**(Suppl):152–60.

13 Richards R, Fowler C, Simpson SF, Renwick AG, Holgate ST. Deep inspiration increases the absorption of inhaled sodium chromoglycate. *Br J Clin Pharmacol* 1989;**27**:861–5.

14 Vaisman N, Koren G, Goldstein D *et al.* Pharmacokinetics of inhaled salbutamol in patients with cystic fibrosis versus healthy young adults. *J Pediatr* 1987;**111**:914–17.

15 Conte JE, Upton RA, Phelps RT *et al.* Use of a specific and sensitive assay to determine pentamidine pharmacokinetics in patients with AIDS. *J Infect Dis* 1986;**154**:923–9.

16 Donnelly H, Bernard EM, Rothkotter H, Gold JWM, Armstrong D. Distribution of pentamidine in patients with AIDS. *J Infect Dis* 1988;**157**:985–9.

17 Conte JE, Golden JA. Concentration of aerosolised pentamidine in bronchoalveolar lavage, systemic absorption and excretion. *Antimicrob Agents Chemother* 1988;**32**:1490–3.

18 Girard PM, Clair B, Certain A *et al.* Comparison of plasma concentrations of aerosolized pentamidine in non-ventilated and ventilated patients with pneumocystosis. *Am Rev Respir Dis* 1989;**140**:1607–10.

19 Kremer JMH, Wilting J, Janssen LHM. Drug binding to human alpha-1-acid glycoprotein in health and disease. *Pharmacol Rev* 1988;**40**:1–47.

20 Paxton JW, Briant RH. Alpha1-acid glycoprotein concentrations and propranolol binding in elderly patients with acute illness. *Br J Clin Pharmacol* 1984;**18**:806–10.

21 Zarowitz BJ, Shlom J, Eichenhorn MS, Popovich J. Alterations in theophylline protein binding in acutely ill patients with COPD. *Chest* 1985;**87**:766–9.

22 Vallner JJ, Speir WA, Kolbeck RC, Harrison GN, Bransome ED. Effect of pH on the binding of theophylline to serum proteins. *Am Rev Respir Dis* 1979;**120**:83–6.

23 Bergogne-Berezin E. Pharmacokinetics of antibiotics in respiratory secretions. In: Pennington E, ed. *Respiratory infections: diagnosis and management.* New York: Raven Press, 1983:461–79.

24 Barza M, Cuchural G. General principles of antibiotic tissue penetration. *J Antimicrob Chemother* 1985;**15**(Suppl):59–75.

25 Wise R. The clinical relevance of protein binding and tissue concentrations in antimicrobial therapy. *Clin Pharmacokinet* 1986;**11**:470–82.

26 De Groot R, Smith AL. Antibiotic pharmacokinetics in cystic fibrosis: differences and clinical significance. *Clin Pharmacokinet* 1987;**13**:228–53.

27 Zarowitz BJ, Pancorbo S, Dubey J, Wadenstorer F, Popovich J. Variability in theophylline volume of distribution and clearance in patients with acute respiratory failure requiring mechanical ventilation. *Chest* 1988;**93**:379–85.

28 Arnold JD, Hill GN, Sansom LN. A comparison of the pharmacokinetics of theophylline in asthmatic children in the acute episode and in remission. *Eur J Clin Pharmacol* 1981;**20**:443–7.

29 Farrell GC. Drug metabolism in extrahepatic disease. *Pharmacol Ther* 1987;**35**:375–404.

30 Perkins MW, Dasta JF, De Haven B. Physiologic implications of mechanical ventilation on pharmacokinetics. *DICP* 1989;**23**:316–23.

31 Roth RA, Wiersma DA. Role of the lung in total body clearance of circulating drugs. *Clin Pharmacokinet* 1979;**4**:355–67.

32 Au WYW, Dutt AR, De Soyza N. Theophylline knietics in chronic obstructive airways disease in the elderly. *Clin Pharmacol Ther* 1985;**37**:472–8.

33 Gillis CN, Pitt BR, Wiedemann HP, Hammond GL. Depressed prostaglandin E1 and 5-hydroxytryptamine removal in patients with adult respiratory distress syndrome. *Am Rev Respir Dis* 1986;**134**:739–44.

34 Morel DR, Dargent F, Bachmann M, Suter PM, Junod AF. Pulmonary extraction of serotonin and propranolol in patients with adult respiratory distress syndrome. *Am Rev Respir Dis* 1985;**132**:479–84.

35 Triginer C, Fernandez I, Rello J, Benito S. Gentamicin pharmacokinetic changes related to mechanical ventilation. *Ann Pharmacother* 1989;**23**:923–4.

36 Richard C, Berdeaux A, Delion F *et al.* Effect of mechanical ventilation on hepatic drug pharmacokinetics. *Chest* 1986;**90**:837–41.

156

37 Sarrubi FA, Hull JH. Amikacin serum concentrations: prediction of levels and dosage guidelines. *Ann Intern Med* 1978;**89**:612–18.

38 Kirby MG, Dasta JF, Armstrong DK, Tallman R. Effect of low dose dopamine on the pharmacokinetics of tobramycin in dogs. *Antimicrob Agents Chemother* 1986;**29**:168–70.

39 Garrett ER. Pharmacokinetics and clearances related to renal processes. *Int J Clin Pharmacol* 1978;**16**:155–72.

40 Levy G, Koysooko R. Renal clearance of theophylline in man. *J Clin Pharmacol* 1976;**16**:329–32.

41 Contrepois A, Brion N, Garaud JJ *et al.* Renal disposition of gentamicin, dibekacin, tobramycin, netilmycin and maikacin in humans. *Antimicrob Agents Chemother* 1985;**27**:520–4.

42 Kaplan LD, Jones D, Aw TY, Rudman D. Oxygen dependence of acetaminophen metabolism. *Am Rev Respir Dis* 1983;**127**(Suppl):292.

43 Woodroffe AJM, Bayliss MK, Park GR. The effects of hypoxia on drug-metabolising enzymes. *Drug Metab Rev* 1995;**27**:471–95.

44 Arias IM, Jakoby WB, Popper H, Schachter D, Shafritz DA. *The liver, biology and pathobiology*, 2nd edn. New York; Raven Press, 1988.

45 Angus PW, Morgan DJ, Smallwood RA. Review article: hypoxia and hepatic drug metabolism–clinical implications. *Aliment Pharmacol Ther* 1990;**4**:213–25.

46 Aw TY, Jones DP. Secondary bioenergetic hypoxia. Inhibition of sulfation and glucuronidation reactionsin isolated hepatocytes at low O_2 concentrations. *J Biol Chem* 1982;**257**:8997–9007.

47 Jones DP. Hypoxia and drug metabolism. *Biochem Pharmacol* 1981;**30**:1019–23.

48 Jones DP, Mason HS. Gradients of O_2 concentration in hepatocytes. *J Biol Chem* 1978;**253**:4874–80.

49 Smith BR, Born JL, Garcia DJ. Influence of hypoxia on the metabolism and excretion of misonidazole by the isolated perfused rat liver – a model system. *Biochem Pharmacol* 1983;**32**:1609–12.

50 Angus PW, Mihaly GW, Morgan DJ, Smallwood RA. Oxygen dependence of omeprazole clearance and the production of its sulphone and sulphide metabolites in the isolated perfused rat liver. *J Pharmacol Exp Ther* 1989;**250**:1043–7.

51 Park GR, Pichard L, Tinel M *et al.* What changes drug metabolism in critically ill patients? Two preliminary studies in isolated hepatocytes. *Anaesthesia* 1994;**49**:188–91.

52 Merritt JH, Medina MA. Altitude-induced alterations in drug action and metabolism. *Life Sci* 1968;**7**:1163–9.

53 Hawkins SF, Hankinson JB, Merritt JH, Medina MM. Effect of reduced barometric pressure on drug action and metabolism in mice. *Biochem Pharmacol* 1971;**20**:2221–9.

54 Baumel I, De Feo JJ, Lal H. Alterations in brain sensitivity and barbiturate metabolism unrelated to aggression in socially deprived mice. *Psychopharmacologica* 1970;**18**:320–4.

55 Roth RA, Rubin RJ. Comparison of the effect of carbon monoxide and of hypoxic hypoxia. II Hexobarbital metabolism in the isolated perfused liver. *J Pharmacol Exp Ther* 1976;**199**:61–6.

56 Mustala OO, Azarnoff DL. Effect of oxygen tension on drug levels and pharmacological action in the intact animal. *Proc Soc Exp Biol Med* 1969;**132**:37–41.

57 Aw TY, Shan X, Sillau AH, Jones DP. Effect of chronic hypoxia on acetaminophen metabolism in the rat. *Biochem Pharmacol* 1991;**42**:1029–38.

58 Shan X, Aw TY, Smith ER *et al.* Effect of hypoxia on detoxication enzymes in rat liver. *Biochem Pharmacol* 1992;**43**:2421–6.

59 Berry LJ. General summary of the anthrax conference. *Fed Proc* 1967;**26**:1569–70.

60 Longmuir IS, Pashko L. The induction of cytochrome P-450 by hypoxia. *Adv Exp Med Biol* 1976;**75**:171–5.

61 Jones DP, Aw TY, Shan X. Drug metabolism and toxicity during hypoxia. *Drug Metab Rev* 1989;**20**:247–60.

62 Miller E, Park GR. The effect of oxygen on propofol-induced inhibition of microsomal cytochrome P450 3A4. *Anaesthesia* 1999;**54**:320–2.

63 Jones DP. Renal metabolism during normoxia, hypoxia, and ischemic injury. *Annu Rev Physiol* 1986;**48**:33–50.

64 Nellimarkka O, Niinikoski J. Oxygen and carbon dioxide tensions in the canine kidney during arterial occlusion and hemmorhagic hypotension. *Surg Gynecol Obstet* 1984;**158**:27–32.

10: Children

ROBERT C TASKER

The aim of drug therapy in children is to produce a desired and predictable pharmacological response, while also minimising the occurrence of unwanted side effects. It is not possible to achieve this goal by merely extrapolating pharmacokinetic and pharmacodynamic data from adults to children: there is more to development than a change in mass and volume. In Chapter 2 the effect of underlying disease, stress, temperature, level of nutrition, and organ-system dysfunction on drug absorption, distribution, metabolism, and elimination were described with particular reference to intensive care practice. An added dimension, however, is the significance of ageing and what effect this factor may have on pharmacology. In this context, much of what we know is derived from healthy adult volunteers, which – as already stated – may not be appropriate when considering treatment at the extremes of age. This chapter therefore highlights one aspect of the problem: the young and the effect of postnatal development and infancy on pharmacokinetics, specifically drug absorption, distribution, metabolism, and excretion.

Age and drug absorption

Development, or age, may influence the extent or rate at which a drug is absorbed into the systemic circulation. For oral or nasogastric drug administration such age-related factors include: changes in anatomy, for example, the surface area available for absorption; changes in functional state, for example, gastric and duodenal pH; changes in physiology, for example, gastric emptying time, bile salt pool size; and changes due to extrauterine adaptation, for example, bacterial colonisation of the gastrointestinal tract.[1,2] When treating the very young, the potential influence of each of these factors needs to be considered. However, surprisingly, adult values in gastric pH and emptying,[3-5] and in pancreatic exocrine function[6,7] may be achieved at quite a young age (Table 10.1).

Age and drug distribution

After a drug is absorbed into the systemic circulation it can be distributed throughout the whole body. The magnitude of a drug's apparent volume of

Table 10.1   Development and factors affecting absorption of orally administered drugs.

Factor	Age when adult values are reached
Gastric acid secretion	3 months
The neonate has relative achlorhydria which results in increased bioavailability of basic drugs	
Gastric emptying	6–8 months
Prolonged emptying in the infant, particularly when stressed, will reduce or delay the peak concentration of orally administered drugs	
Exocrine pancreatic function	9–12 months
Relative insufficiency in infancy will decrease the bioavailability of oral agents where intra-luminal hydrolysis is required before absorption of the parent drug	

distribution (V_d) provides some information on where the drug is distributed as well as on what might be the optimal dosage regimen for achieving a specific therapeutic concentration (see Chapter 2). Several factors such as plasma protein concentration and tissue binding will affect the V_d, where the relationship is expressed by the equation:

$$V_d = V_b + V_t(f_B/f_T)$$

where V_b is blood volume, V_t is tissue volume, f_B is fraction of unbound drug in the blood, and f_T is the fraction of unbound drug in tissue.[2] Since age influences the composition and size of the body's compartments, as well as any drug–protein binding characteristics, it can be concluded that a drug's V_d is age dependent.

Body compartments and age

The absolute amount of body water and fat depend on age.[8,9] Major changes in the body's water content and its compartments occur in the first year of life; thereafter these values approach adult proportions (Table 10.2). During the first year of life there is a rapid decrease in the relative volumes of total body water and of extracellular water. Afterwards, there is a smaller decrease in the volume of extracellular water. With regard to body fat, the percentage of body weight that is composed of fat is approximately 15% at birth, and then 20% at six months of age, before it begins to fall gradually to adolescent proportions over the following years.

Protein binding and age

Drug binding to plasma proteins depends on a number of age-related variables:[10] first, the absolute quantity of protein available; second, the number of available protein-binding sites; and third, the affinity constant of

Table 10.2   The ontogeny of water distribution.

Age	TBW	% total body weight ECF	ICF
Birth	75	35–45	33
6 months	60	~25	37
12 months	60	25–30	40
Puberty	60	~20	40
Adult	50–60	~20	40

ECF, extracellular fluid; ICF, intracellular fluid; TBW, total body water.
Adapted from[2].

the drug for the proteins. Changes in all of these factors will have significant bearing on the design of optimal dosage regimens. (They also indicate the folly of applying adult-defined serum concentration–effect relationships to pharmacotherapy in young infants.) For example, there are important differences in the binding of ampicillin, benzylpenicillin, phenobarbitone, and phenytoin to plasma proteins in neonatal plasma when compared with the binding in adult plasma.[11] Greater concentrations of free drug are to be found in the blood samples from infants.[12] In this context, it should also be noted that, at any age, a drug's V_d and clearance will be influenced by the extent to which it is bound to albumin, α_1-acid glycoprotein, or lipoprotein. The serum albumin and total protein concentration are decreased during infancy, and they only approach adult values by the age of 10–12 months.[11] Similarly, the level of α_1-acid glycoprotein undergoes an ontogeny: adult levels are reached by 12 months of age, from a level at birth which is about one-third of that found in adults.

Age and drug metabolism

The overall rate of drug removal from the body is comprised of its metabolic biotransformation in the liver, its elimination in stool or urine, and its exhalation via the lungs. This section addresses the ontogenic aspects of hepatic drug clearance, which is perhaps the most significant, developmentally, of all the above routes of clearance, although, of course, age-related changes in respiratory rate, tidal volume, and minute ventilation should not be underestimated, particularly when administering inhalational anaesthetics.

The liver is a major organ even in the infant: the relative weight of the liver as a proportion of total body weight at birth and in adulthood is 5% and 2%, respectively.[13] Hepatic drug clearance depends on hepatic blood flow, free-drug concentration, hepatic uptake and metabolism, and biliary excretion. The hepatic clearance of a drug can be expressed as:

$$Cl_h = \frac{f_B \times Cl_{int}}{Q \times Q + (f_B \times Cl_{int})}$$

where Cl_h is hepatic clearance, Q is hepatic blood flow, f_B is the fraction of free drug, and Cl_{int} is the free intrinsic clearance, which is a measure of hepatocellular metabolism.[2] From the equation it is evident that drugs mainly cleared from the body by the liver can be flow or capacity limited, that is, they depend on the degree of hepatic uptake and metabolism. Flow-limited drugs have a high extraction ratio and a high Cl_{int} in relation to hepatic blood flow. By contrast, capacity-limited drugs have a low extraction ratio and low Cl_{int}. Also, it is apparent that hepatic clearance of capacity-limited drugs may be influenced, in some instances, by protein binding: for drugs that have extraction ratios which approach free-drug concentration, hepatic clearance will be increased by a decrease in the extent of protein binding. For drugs that have extraction ratios that are much less than the free-drug concentration, this phenomenon will not occur: hepatic clearance will remain a function of Cl_{int}. From this description, one can infer how age or maturity might influence developmental differences in drug metabolism. For example, the ontogeny of hepatic blood flow, protein-binding characteristics, and hepatocellular drug-metabolising enzyme activities. In regard to the latter, there are significant changes which are discussed below.

Drug biotransformation: genotype and development

As already described in Chapter 2, the hepatic biotransformation reactions are classified into two main types: phase I and phase II. The phase I reactions, which include oxidation, reduction, or hydrolysis, introduce or reveal a functional group within the drug. The phase II reaction results in a further increase in the polarity of this metabolic intermediate by conjugation with endogenous sulphate, acetate, glucuronic acid, glutathione, or glycine (a physicochemical step essential for renal excretion). With regard to the relationship between development and drug biotransformation, it should be noted that many of the enzymes responsible for drug biotransformation are polymorphically expressed.[14,15] This phenomenon would mean that, genetically, adults may be anywhere on a spectrum which ranges from fast to slow metabolisers. At birth, infants may be phenotypically slow metabolisers for certain drug-metabolising pathways, only acquiring a phenotype consistent with their genotype, at a later time, on maturity.

In human drug metabolism, the most important of the phase I haem-thiolate P450s (cytochromes P450s) are found in the CYP 1, CYP 2, and CYP 3 gene families. With regard to the phase II enzymes, several are polymorphically expressed, including glutathione S-transferase μ,[16] arylamine N-acetyltransferases (NAT 1 and NAT 2),[17] catechol O-methyltransferase,[18] and thiopurine S-methyltransferase (TPMT);[19] and of these, in children, NAT 2 and TPMT are particularly important. When considering the ontogeny of drug-metabolising activity, there are, however, more complex issues, besides individual enzyme activity, which may be at play. For example, specific enzyme activity can follow a specific developmental pattern (Table 10.3), but overall drug biotransformation capacity may, in fact, represent a composite or combination of these individual drug-metabolising enzyme activities.[14]

161

Table 10.3   The ontogeny of drug-metabolising enzymes.

Enzyme	Substrate examples	Ontogeny of activity
Phase 1		
CYP 1A2	Caffeine, theophylline	4 months: adult value 1–2 years: >adult value Puberty: adult competence
CYP 2C19	Diazepam, phenytoin, propranolol	1 week: low value 6 months: adult value 3–4 years: 1·5–1·8 times adult Puberty: adult competence
CYP 2C9	Phenytoin, diclofenac	1 week: low value 6 months: adult value 3–4 years: 1·5–1·8 times adult Puberty: adult competence
CYP 2D6	Flecanide, propranolol ondansetron, cisapride, dextromethorphan	1 week: present 1 month: 20% adult value 3–5 years: adult competence
CYP 3A4	Midazolam, cyclosporin, tacrolimus, nifedipine, carbamazepine, cisapride	1 month: low activity 6–12 months: adult value 1–4 years: >adult value Puberty: adult competence
Phase II		
NAT 2	Clonazepam, spironolactone, sulphamethoxazole	2 months: slow phenotype 4–6 months: adult phenotype 1–3 years: adult competence
TMPT	Captopril, azathioprine	Birth: >adult value 7–9 years: adult competence

Adapted from[14].

By way of illustration of this phenomenon, the developmental aspects of various phase I and phase II enzymes are now discussed. Much of this information has been derived from studies using drugs as "probes" to reveal age-dependent differences. For example, first, for cytochrome P450 1A2, using caffeine 3-demethylation as the probe, activity is very low in neonates and matures to adult values by about 4 months of postnatal age.[20] Second, for cytochrome P450 2D6 activity, using dextromethorphan O-demethylation to dextrorphan as the probe, 2–9% of children are poor metabolisers,[21,22] which is similar to adults,[23] and by the age of 10 years, adult catalytic activity is present.[22] Third, for cytochrome P450 2C19, using the 4'-hydroxylation of the S-enantiomer of mephenytoin as the probe,[24] 3–5% of whites and 20% of Asians have mephenytoin hydroxylase deficiency;[22] and, using phenytoin disposition, activity comparable to adults is reached by six months of age. Higher than adult activity is present between 3 and 4 years of age, but this activity then declines to adult values by the end of puberty.[25] Fourth, for cytochrome P450 2C9, using phenytoin biotransformation to the parahydroxide metabolite, adult activity is gained by six months of age, with levels above this value by 3–10 years of age, which then, like cytochrome P450 2C19 activity, declines back to the adult value by the completion of puberty.[25] Last, for cytochrome P450 3A4, using the biotransformation of carbamazepine to its 10,11-epoxide metabolite as the probe, children have higher activity which subsequently declines gradually to adult values.[26,27]

The phase II enzymes also have varying ontogenies with different developmental profiles. For example, dependent on race, 5–90% of the adult population are phenotypically slow metabolisers with regard to NAT 2 activity.[23,28] Ontogenetically, using oral caffeine administration and quantification of the 1-methylxanthine ratio in urine as the probe, all infants between 1 and 2 months of age are phenotypically slow acetylators, by 4–8 months of age 50% are fast acetylators, and by 8 months to 1 year of age 62% are fast acetylators.[29] Adult-like population proportions in NAT 2 activity are fully expressed by 3 years of age.[21] TPMT activity is high in almost 90% of the population and intermediate in just over 10%.[30] Developmentally, peripheral blood TPMT activity in infants is higher than that found in adults, with adult activity being reached between 7 and 9 years of age.[31,32]

Age and drug excretion

Renal function is vital for the excretion of many drugs and their water-soluble metabolites. The factors which are important in this process are glomerular filtration rate (GFR), renal blood flow, and the extent of drug protein binding. Each of these is influenced by growth and development. For example, although there may be some variation attributable to maturation at birth,[33] GFR is 2–4 ml/min in full-term infants, 8–20 ml/min in 3-day-old infants, and approaches adult values by 3–5 months of age.[33,34] With regard to renal blood flow, there are increases occurring with age which may be due to maturation, or changes in cardiac output, or a reduction in peripheral vascular resistance.[35,36] At birth, the kidneys receive only 5% of the cardiac output compared with 15–20% seen in adults. This translates into a renal blood flow of about 12 ml/min in infancy, with adult values being attained by 1 year of age.[1,36] Last, protein binding effects the amount of drug filtered: the amount filtered is inversely related to the degree of protein binding. Developmental aspects of drug–protein interaction have been discussed above.

Conclusion

The above review hopefully exemplifies the importance of considering drug administration in the developing human as distinct from the characteristics of administration in adults. When planning treatment, children cannot be thought of as small adults. In fact, there are major developmental changes which means that when dealing with children one should ask what is the impact of age and development on:

- absorption of oral or nasogastric administered drug
- body compartment size and proportions
- drug–protein binding
- the amount and activity of constitutively expressed metabolising enzymes
- renal function.

Taken together, it is clear that if a new drug is to be used in critically ill children, then paediatric-specific pharmacokinetic and pharmacodynamic data should be a prerequisite of such practice.

1 Besunder JB, Reed MD, Blumer JL. Principles of drug biodisposition in the neonate: a critical evaluation of the pharmacokinetic–pharmacokinetic interface. *Clin Pharmacokinet* 1988;**14**:189–286.
2 Reed MD, Besunder JB. Developmental pharmacology: ontogenic basis of drug disposition. *Pediatr Clin North Am* 1989;**36**:1053–74.
3 Agunod M, Yomaguchi N, Lopez R, Luhby AL, Glass GB. Correlative study of hydrochloric acid, pepsin and intrinsic factor secretion in newborns and infants. *Am J Dig Dis* 1969;**14**:400–14.
4 Hyman PE, Feldman EJ, Ament ME, Byrne WJ, Euler AR. Effect of external feeding on the maintenance of gastric acid secretory function. *Gastroenterology* 1983;**84**:341–5.
5 Gupta M, Brans YW. Gastric retention in neonates. *Pediatrics* 1978;**62**:26–9.
6 Hadorn B, Zoppi G, Shmerling DH, Prader A, McIntyre I, Anderson CM. Quantitative assessment of exocrine pancreatic function in infants and children. *J Pediatr* 1968;**73**:39–50.
7 Zoppi G, Andreotti G, Pajno-Ferraru F, Njai DM, Gaburro D. Exocrine pancreatic function in premature and full-term neonates. *Pediatr Res* 1972;**6**:880–6.
8 Friis-Hansen B. Body water compartments in children: changes during growth and related changes in composition. *Pediatrics* 1961;**28**:168–81.
9 Friis-Hansen B. Water distribution in the foetus and the newborn infant. *Acta Paediatr Scand* 1983;**305**:7–11.
10 Pacifici GM, Viani A, Taddeucci-Brunelli T, Rizzo G, Carrai M, Schulz HU. Effects of development, aging, and renal and hepatic insufficiency as well as hemodialysis on the plasma concentration of albumin and α_1-acid glycoprotein: implications for binding of drugs. *Ther Drug Monitor* 1986;**8**:259–63.
11 Ehrnebo M, Agurell S, Jalling B, Boreus LO. Age difference in drug binding by plasma proteins: studies in human fetuses, neonates and adults. *J Clin Pharmacol* 1971;**3**:189–93.
12 Kurz H, Mauser-Ganshorn A, Stickel HH. Differences in the binding of drugs to plasma proteins from newborn and adult man. I. *Eur J Clin Pharmacol* 1977;**11**:463–7.
13 Boreus LO. *Principles of pediatric pharmacology*. New York: Churchill Livingstone, 1982 : 48.
14 Leeder JS, Kearns GL. Pharmacogenetics in pediatrics: implications for practice. *Pediatr Clin North Am* 1997;**44**:55–77.
15 Bailey DS, Bondar A, Furness LM. Pharmacogenomics – it's not just pharmacogenetics. *Curr Opinion Biotech* 1998;**9**:595–601.
16 Seidegaard J, Vorachek WR, Pero RW, Pearson WR. Hereditary differences in the expression of the human glutathione transferase active on trans-stilbene oxide are due to gene deletion. *Proc Natl Acad Sci USA* 1988;**85**:7293–7.
17 Weber WW, Hein DW. *N*-Acetylation pharmacogenetics. *Pharmacol Rev* 1985;**37**:25–79.
18 Lundstrom K, Tenhunen J, Tilgmann C, Karliunen T, Panula P, Ulmanen I. Cloning, expression and structure of catechol-*O*-methyltransferase. *Biochem Biophys Acta* 1995;**1251**:1–10.
19 Krynetski EY, Tai H-L, Yates CR *et al.* Genetic polymorphism of thiopurine *S*-methyltransferase: clinical importance and molecular mechanisms. *Pharmacogenetics* 1996;**6**:279–90.
20 Cazeneuve C, Pons G, Rey E *et al.* Biotransformation of caffeine in human liver microsomes from foetuses, neonates, infants and adults. *Br J Pharmacol* 1994;**37**:405–12.

21 Evans WE, Relling MV, Petros WP, Meyer WH, Mirro J, Crow WR. Dextromethorphan and caffeine as probes for simultaneous determination of debrisoquin-oxidation and *N*-acetylation phenotypes in children. *Clin Pharmacol Ther* 1989;**45**:568–73.

22 Relling MV, Cherrie J, Schell MJ, Petros WP, Meyer WH, Evans WE. Lower prevalence of the debrisoquin oxidative poor metabolizer phenotype in American black versus white subjects. *Clin Pharmacol Ther* 1991;**50**:308–13.

23 May DG. Genetic differences in drug disposition. *J Clin Pharmacol* 1994;**34**:881–97.

24 Goldstein JA, Faletto MB, Romkes-Sparks M *et al.* Evidence that CYP2C19 is the major (*S*)-mephenytoin 4'-hydroxylase in humans. Biochemistry 1994;**33**:1743–52.

25 Dodson WE. Special pharmacokinetic considerations in children. *Epilepsia* 1987;**28**(S1):S56–70.

26 Kroetz DL, Kerr BM, McFarland LV, Loiseau P, Wilensky AJ, Levy RH. Measurement of in vivo microsomal epoxide hydrolase activity in white subjects. *Clin Pharmacol Ther* 1993;**53**:306–15.

27 Korinthenberg R, Haug C, Hannak D. The metabolization of carbamazepine to CBZ-10,11-epoxide in children from the newborn age to adolescence. *Neuropediatrics* 1994;**25**:214–16.

28 Meyer UA. Genetic polymorphisms of drug metabolism. *Fundam Clin Pharmacol* 1990;**4**:595–615.

29 Pariente-Khayat A, Pons G, Rey E *et al.* Caffeine acetylator phenotying during maturation in infants. *Pediatr Res* 1991;**29**:492–5.

30 McLeod HL, Relling MV, Liu Q, Piu CH, Evans WE. Polymorphic thiopurine methyltransferase activity in erythrocytes is indicative of activity in leukemic blasts from children with acute lymphoblastic leukemia. *Blood* 1995;**85**:1897–902.

31 McLeod HL, Krynetski EY, Williams JA, Evans WE. Higher activity of polymorphic thiopurine *S*-methyltransferase in erythrocytes from neonates compared to adults. *Pharmacogenetics* 1995;**5**:281–6.

32 Park-Hah JO, Klemetsdal B, Lysaa R, Choi KH, Aarbakke J. Thiopurine methyltransferase activity in Korean population sample of children. *Clin Pharmacol Ther* 1996;**60**:68–74.

33 Arant BS. Developmental patterns of renal functional maturation compared in the human neonate. *J Pediatr* 1978;**92**:705–12.

34 Leake RD, Trygstad CW. Glomerular filtration rate during the period of adaptation to extrauterine life. *Pediatr Res* 1977;**11**:959–62.

35 Hook JB, Bailie MD. Perinatal renal pharmacology. *Annu Rev Pharmacol Toxicol* 1979;**19**:491–509.

36 West JR, Smith HW, Chasis H. Glomerular filtration rate, effective renal blood flow and maximal tubular excretory capacity in infancy. *J Pediatr* 1948;**32**:10–18.

11: Safe drug prescribing in the critically ill

ROBIN J WHITE, GILBERT PARK

A doctor's responsibilities when prescribing for a critically ill patient are no different from those when prescribing for ordinary patients. In its introduction, the British National Formulary advises doctors that: "Medicines should only be prescribed when they are necessary, and in all cases the benefits of administering the medicine should be considered in relation to the risk involved."[1] The aim of this chapter is to summarise many of the points raised elsewhere in the book, and to offer some advice on how the risks of drug prescription can be minimised in this group of patients.

Under normal circumstances, a doctor would be expected to be in possession of a full medical history, the results of clinical examination and appropriate laboratory investigations. In the critically ill, full information may not be available. Drug allergy is another area in which vital information may not be available in emergency situations. All treatment except that which is immediately necessary should be delayed until further information can be obtained from relatives, general practitioners, or previous medical notes. Questions to be considered before prescribing a drug would include:

- Is it really necessary?
- What are the indications, contraindications, and side effects of the proposed treatment?
- Are there any safer, cheaper, or alternative treatments available for this condition?
- If treatment is not urgent, can further information be obtained before prescribing which would make the prescription safer?

Critically ill patients differ from other patients in terms of both their pharmacodynamic responses to drugs and their pharmacokinetic handling of drugs. An understanding of these differences will enable doctors to prescribe more appropriately, and more safely, for this group of patients.

Is drug treatment really necessary?

For many doctors, the initial response to illness is to prescribe. After all, it is what the patients, their relatives, and their attendants often expect. But

166

there are many situations in which non-drug treatments should be considered in the first instance, for example, resuscitation of a patient who has collapsed with a supraventricular tachycardia. The following drug treatments might be considered:

- verapamil – is this patient is taking β-blockers? If so, the result could be an irretrievable asystolic arrest.[2,3]
- adenosine – is this patient asthmatic? Adenosine may precipitate severe acute asthma.[2,3]
  The following non-drug treatments might also be considered:
- carotid massage[4]
- ocular massage[5] – although this may cause retinal damage
- forced expiration against a closed glottis (Valsalva manoeuvre)[5]
- synchronised DC cardioversion[6]
- stopping drug treatments that might be causing the arrhythmia, such as dopamine.

In circumstances where the patient's medical and drug history is unknown, the use of non-pharmacological interventions can avoid the risks of pharmacological treatment. If these manoeuvres fail, and the patient remains hypotensive, the relative risk of drug treatment decreases as the risk of not treating increases.

What are the indications?

In most countries, each drug has a list of licensed indications. If drugs are administered outside these indications, any complications which arise from the use of that drug will not be the liability of the manufacturer, but usually of the doctor.

Before prescribing any drug, a doctor has to be satisfied that the drug is both necessary and appropriate. For any doctor to know the detailed pharmacokinetics and pharmacodynamics of every drug likely to be prescribed is unrealistic. To simplify and standardise treatment, many ICUs have produced treatment algorithms and guidelines for the commonly encountered conditions. Algorithms are defined as sets of rules used for problem solving. They usually start with a diagnosis being made. The doctor is then guided through stepwise decisions to arrive finally at the recommended therapeutic treatment for the set of circumstances currently faced.

Treatment guidelines are usually didactic, based on "If the diagnosis is X, the treatment is Y and Z." One produced for use internationally is shown in Figure 11.1, whilst a more local one takes the form of a list of instructions as shown in Box 11.1.

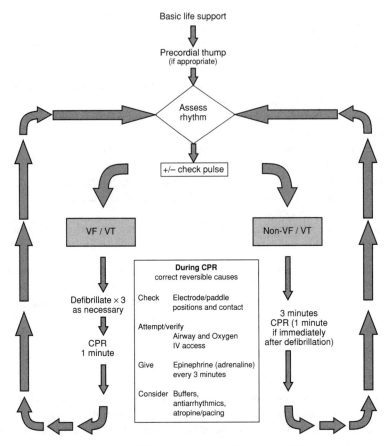

Figure 11.1   Adult advanced life support algorithms. Guidelines for the management of life-threatening arrhythmias.[1]

Box 11.1 Guidelines for terminal weaning on an intensive care unit

Aim: To ensure that terminally ill patients receiving mechanical ventilation die with dignity and without suffering.

Guidelines:

1. The patient's condition is reviewed by the referring clinician and the available ICU consultants. They must all agree that further treatment is hopeless. The nursing staff are involved in these discussions.
2. An Intensive Care consultant and a nurse will discuss the patient's prognosis with the relatives. Normally the fact that the patient is hopelessly ill is introduced to them over one or more days. This gives relatives time to come to terms with the situation. The consultant and the nurse will also explain the way in which treatment will be withdrawn.
3. The Intensive Care consultant records the decision to withdraw treatment in the patient's notes. He also documents:
   - his discussion with the family
   - specific instructions for terminal care.
4. The nurse will separately record all discussions and decisions in the nursing notes.
5. The patient is sedated to ensure that he/she is comfortable. Analgesia is given if necessary to ensure that the patient is pain free.
6. Infusions of vasoactive drugs are stopped. All other prescriptions, e.g. antibiotics, are cancelled.
7. Respiratory support is withdrawn:
   - Providing muscle relaxants have not been given to the patient, the ventilator mode is changed to SIMV and the SIMV rate is halved every 30 minutes.
   - If the patient is able to breathe spontaneously, the trachea is extubated.
8. Appropriate monitoring of the patient will continue. This may include measurement of arterial blood gases or plasma concentrations of potassium. This may allow more accurate predictions to be made about when the patient may die.
9. The patient's family is given as much privacy as possible. It may be appropriate to transfer the dying patient to a side room, or possibly a general ward if he/she is likely to survive for more than 24 hours. It is usually preferable to allow the patient to die in the ICU where the family can be offered support by familiar members of staff. The support of religious and/or cultural organisations may be sought.
10. All nursing and medical actions are carefully recorded.
11. Staff may find terminal care of patients with whom they have been closely associated stressful and distressing. It is important to seek support and guidance of colleagues and other professionals such as the hospital chaplain.

Local guidelines directing prescribing usually result from senior staff looking at all the available evidence, and producing a consensus view. Clearly, such views will vary from unit to unit. They provide a means by which senior staff can guide the care delivered by their junior and nursing staff without having to be personally present on the unit 24 hours a day.

In a similar way, guidelines and algorithms may be produced nationally. Some algorithms, such as the life support algorithms published by the Resuscitation Council (UK), which are based on the ILCOR Advisory Statement, are adopted in most hospitals. Nationwide adoption of such algorithms allows direct comparison of the results of different units. It also generates data on a large number of patients, which is turn allows better assessment of the algorithm, and facilitates subsequent changes to it if evidence becomes available which changes the consensus view. Some people would argue, however, that the use of algorithms and protocols take much of the intellectual challenge out of medicine, and make it harder for new innovations to come about. Fear that deviation from the accepted protocols will leave an individual doctor open to criticism from others should their therapies prove to be less effective than those prescribed in algorithms and protocols already in use may deter the development of novel therapeutic strategies and the development of new drugs.

Guidelines and protocols

Guidelines are produced to guide prescribing or treatment and, as such, are only guidelines. They are there to guide those with less experience. Practitioners with sufficient knowledge and experience can make their own alternative decisions provided they can justify their decisions. Protocols, however, tend to be stricter and allow less freedom. They are pre-prescribed interventions for a particular condition or set of circumstances. In such circumstances, failure to follow recognised protocols leaves a doctor or nurse open to criticism. Protocols have the advantage that everyone knows what is expected of them. They are usually the result of detailed study, are the recommendations of leading experts, and are generally accepted as current best advice on the situations that they cover. However, it has been argued that the issuing of such didactic statements deters individuals from trying novel therapies and interventions because of the fear of criticism should their attempt be unsuccessful.

What are the contraindications and side effects?

These two headings will be dealt with together because they are both based around pharmacokinetic and pharmacodynamic considerations. An understanding of these two basic building blocks of pharmacology will allow careful consideration of each prescription, and thereby minimise the potential for harm because of inappropriate drug use in critically ill patient groups.

Absorption

The first important point to remember is that formulation is important. This refers to the physical form in which the drug is presented. Many drugs are available in short-acting and slow-release formulations. These are potentially dangerous in the critically ill because they are so unpredictable. They may be labelled Continus, CR, LA, MR, SA, SR, or XL. Drugs available in the United Kingdom in this format include:

- antihypertensive agents such as Inderal-LA® and Betaloc SA®
- antianginal drugs such as Tildiem-LA®, Cardene SR®, Syscor MR®
- bronchodilator therapies including Bricanyl SA®, Nuelin SA® and Phyllocontin Continus®.

It is important to note that if a drug intended to be given as a once-a day slow-release preparation is given in the same dose of a standard, shorter-acting preparation, the likely result is overdosage. This is because absorption of the slow-release preparation is spread over many hours. Although the same total dose is administered, the peak plasma concentration will be many times higher if the entire dose is available for absorption at a single point in time.

There are also advantages of slow-release preparations that must not be overlooked, for example, the use of transdermal glyceryl trinitrate (GTN) patches provides effective therapy and can reduce the risks inherent in the intravenous route of administration.

Drug interactions also need to be considered when looking at absorption. There are instances where the presence of one substance in the stomach or gastrointestinal tract will affect the absorption of a second, often unrelated drug. For example, the absorption of oral flucloxacillin is reduced by the presence of food in the gastrointestinal tract. Flucloxacillin should therefore be given at least 30 minutes before ingestion of food.[1,7] Alcohol taken with benzodiazepines will enhance the absorption of benzodiazepines from the gastrointestinal tract and reduce their rate of metabolism, an important fact to know when there is concomitant ingestion of these two substances in attempted suicide and parasuicide.[8]

Another important factor to consider relating to drug absorption is pathophysiological conditions of the gastrointestinal tract. Many drugs taken enterally are absorbed from the upper gastrointestinal tract, and undergo significant first-pass metabolism in the liver, which significantly reduces the amount of the drug reaching the systemic circulation. Any disease process which reduces hepatic blood flow, or the liver's metabolic capacity, will affect the bioavailability of these drugs, which include propranolol,[8] opioids, local anaesthetics, and benzodiazepines.[6] Another important consideration is the administration of drugs that alter the pH of the gastrointestinal tract, particularly the stomach. A low pH will facilitate absorption of neutral and acidic drugs, while inhibiting the uptake of basic drugs.[8] Because of this, changes in gastric pH due to pathology or pharma-

171

cological manipulation can have important effects on drug absorption, bioavailability, and the clinical effect. For these reasons, most drugs are given intravenously to the critically ill.

Distribution

There are two important factors to consider about drug distribution in the critically ill. First, some drugs have a distribution which is pH dependent, and second, with some drugs, changes in protein binding are significant.

Drug penetration of the blood–brain barrier is pH dependent. Ionised molecules are lipophobic, and as such cannot penetrate the phospholipid bilayer. Drugs that are weak acids, such as salicylate[9] and phenobarbitone, are more than 50% ionised at normal blood pH, and hence their penetration of the central nervous system is limited. However, in acidosis, the non-ionised proportion of these drugs increases. This increases penetration of the blood–brain barrier, and central nervous system toxicity becomes a risk.

The free-drug concentration of substances that are more than 90% bound to plasma proteins, or drugs with very small volumes of distribution, are susceptible to changes in critically ill patients. Such drugs include penicillins, cephalosporins, sulphonamides, non-steroidal anti-inflammatory drugs, propranolol, and anticoagulants.[10] Usually, the increase in free drug results in greater clearance. This restores the free-drug concentration to normal. However, if the ability to eliminate is reduced, either by renal or hepatic impairment, then the increased concentration will persist. Factors that might change protein binding include:

- changes in albumin and $\alpha 1$-acid glycoprotein concentration, secondary to catabolism and the acute phase response, reducing the binding capacity of the circulation, and hence increasing the concentration of free drug in the plasma (for example, phenytoin,[11] sodium valproate, and warfarin)
- uraemia, when molecules of urea compete for drug binding sites, resulting in increased plasma concentrations of free drugs (for example, warfarin[12] and sodium valproate)[13]
- changes in free-drug concentration resulting in changes in serum levels of drugs frequently measured in the laboratory. For example, consider a patient who has therapeutic plasma concentrations of phenytoin when taking 100 mg 8-hourly. If that patient then becomes critically ill, the plasma albumin levels decrease. Less drug is then protein bound, and a greater free fraction leads to enhanced metabolism and excretion. The measured plasma concentration of phenytoin will decrease. However, the free-drug concentration (the clinically active part), changes very little. In this situation, total serum concentrations of phenytoin will be reduced, but its clinical effectiveness will remain unaltered. In such circumstances, drug monitoring must be carefully interpreted in the light of the clinical circumstances.

Elimination

Metabolism

The majority of drugs used to treat the critically ill undergo either hepatic metabolism, renal excretion, or both. Any changes in the functional capacity of the liver or kidneys will have consequences on drug metabolism (see Figure 11.2) and excretion. One of the roles of the liver is to convert lipophilic molecules into a more hydrophilic form to facilitate urinary excretion.

Another sometimes forgotten role of the liver is the conversion of inactive precursor drugs into their active form (for example, chloral hydrate and enalapril), or the conversion of drugs with some pharmacological activity into metabolites with even greater activity. Clobazam, whose half-life is 18 hours, has metabolites with half-lives of up to 50 hours.[14] For other drugs, accumulation of toxic metabolites, which are not excreted, can present its own problems, such as the fits caused by accumulation of the main metabolite of pethidine, norpethidine.

Aminophylline has important interactions because of its narrow therapeutic index. Patients taking oral theophylline must not be given the usual intravenous loading dose of 5 mg/kg over the first 20 minutes. Administration of such a loading dose would risk making the patient toxic, resulting in convulsions and arrhythmias.[2] In those with congestive cardiac failure, the half-life of aminophylline is increased, whilst in smokers the half-life is reduced.[3] Because smokers and those with a history of heart failure are commonly those in whom aminophylline therapy is considered, detailed medical histories and a working knowledge of the pharmacokinetics of the drug are essential to ensure safe prescribing.

Drugs themselves are sometimes responsible for alterations in the metabolic processes, which bring about their own inactivation. These include

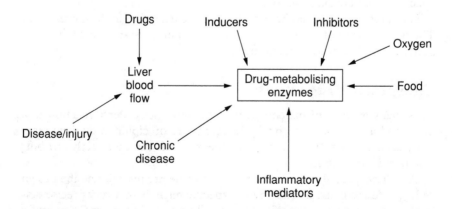

Figure 11.2 Some of the influences on drug-metabolising enzymes.

enzyme induction, particularly of the cytochromes P450. Epileptics on long-term barbiturate therapy or phenytoin, and alcoholics have high levels of some cytochromes, and may rapidly metabolise drugs such as digoxin, cortisol, phenobarbitone, phenytoin, and oral anticoagulants. The result is reduced plasma concentrations, with the need for higher doses to achieve the desired therapeutic effect.[10]

The cytochrome P450 system can also be inhibited by drugs, including cimetidine, chlorpromazine, prednisolone, the oral contraceptive pill, and oral anticoagulants.[14] The reduced metabolism of drugs including pethidine, warfarin, and theophylline, will require their doses to be reduced.

Excretion

The renal tubules filter molecules with a molecular weight of less than 40 000 Da, and so excrete many drugs. If more than 40% of a drug is excreted unchanged in the urine, then changes in renal perfusion and function will result in changes in elimination of the drug, such that doses may need to be adjusted (see Chapter 4).

Active processes are also important in the way the kidneys handle drugs. Digoxin is actively secreted in the distal nephron.[15] This process is also used for excretion of verapamil, spironolactone, and quinidine, which means that coadministration of any of these drugs will reduce excretion of digoxin, and predispose to digoxin toxicity.

Passive processes can also be affected in the critically ill. There is a passive reabsorption of non-ionised drugs from the urine in the collecting ducts. Changes in urinary pH will thus affect drug reabsorption and serum concentrations of many drugs. For weak acids, an acidic urine promotes reabsorption from the collecting duct, and for weak bases, the same happens with an alkaline urine. Drug abusers have exploited this phenomenon for many years. Amphetamine, a weak base, is mixed with baking soda. This alkalinises the urine, resulting in greater reabsorption of the drug from the urine, and a prolonged high from the one dose, thereby maximising the effects and minimising the cost.[10]

The same principle can be used to enhance excretion in drug overdoses. The best example of this is the alkalinisation of urine to trap acid molecules such as salicylate and phenobarbitone.

Unexpected drug effects

As many as 20% of patients in hospital suffer an adverse reaction to a drug, and about 5% of hospital admissions are precipitated by drug reactions. One in every 1000 medical inpatient deaths can be directly attributable to a drug reaction.[5]

Many unexpected drug reactions in medicine are merely classified as an "allergy" to the drug. But allergy is a specific term, with a very precise definition: an allergy is "a specifically induced increased reactivity".[5] Allergies have been classified into four distinct categories. Type I reactions are anaphylaxis, type II are cytotoxic, type III are immune complex mediated, and type IV are delayed-hypersensitivity reactions. In critically ill patients, when immune function is often deranged, anaphylaxis is very rare, and proven allergic reactions are rare. Many patients, when critically ill, will get a rash with drugs that they have taken previously without ill effect, and take again once recovered from their illness without any untoward effects. Thus, in critical illness, there appears to be a loss of discrimination between allergic and non-allergic phenomena.

For many drugs, there is a list of well-known, common side effects that is familiar to most doctors. However, many commonly used drugs have effects that, although much less widely known about, can be of great significance in the care of the critically ill patient. Examples might include the lung damage that can be a result of newer selective serotonin re-uptake inhibitor (SSRI) antidepressant therapy, or coma and fitting as a result of inappropriate antidiuretic hormone (ADH) secretion, which can follow administration of the same class of drugs. Although rare when considered in terms of the total numbers of patients taking these drugs, these causes must be considered when patients present with unusual histories, symptoms, signs, or investigations.

Even drugs commonly used in the ICU, such as opioids, have unexpected effects. Common, widely known side effects, known to the majority of doctors, would include nausea and vomiting, constipation, respiratory depression, and urinary retention. Less well known effects of opiods include:

- Muscle rigidity, which can, on occasions, interfere with mechanical ventilation.
- Bradycardia and hypotension, despite their use in cardiac surgery being based on their cardiovascular stability.
- Morphine which may exacerbate asthma, causing bronchoconstriction and tachycardia as a result of histamine release.
- Fentanyl causing irritation and pruritus, particularly around the nasal region. It is also taken up by the lungs, and as much as 75% of an initial dose undergoes first-pass pulmonary uptake. Saturation of the lungs' storage capacity will result in a change of the pharmacokinetic profile of the drug, and analgesia and respiratory depression may be prolonged.[16]
- Metabolites accumulating in patients receiving infusions. These can cause respiratory depression for up to 7 days after the infusion has been stopped.[17] Other metabolites may also accumulate, but be biologically inactive.[18]
- Pancreatitis.
- Opioids have been shown to have significant effects on the immune system. Chronic morphine administration is often used to induce immunosuppression in laboratory animals. Opioids decrease the proliferation of stimulated lymphocytes, and reduce the production of interferon-α and β.[19] Immune changes vary according to the duration of exposure to opioids. Chronic exposure causes desensitisation of the

175

hypothalamic–pituitary–adrenal axis to the cytokine interleukin-1[20] via central opioid receptors, which can be blocked by naloxone. It has also been shown that interleukin-1, released as part of the stress response, induces opioid receptor expression on endothelial cells, confirming the important interactions of both these systems with the immune system. Acute exposure results in immune suppression mediated by peripheral mechanisms involving the sympathetic nervous system.[21] At a cellular level, morphine has been shown to reduce the amount of growth hormone receptor mRNA in human cultured lymphocytes, and to reduce the binding of 125I-labelled growth hormone to these cells.[22]

- μ opioid receptor stimulation inhibiting tissue protein synthesis. This is attributed to changes in pH and oxygenation secondary to respiratory depression.[23]
- Opioids, which have been shown to affect the secretion of growth hormone from the anterior pituitary,[24] via an action at the hypothalamic level, from where pulsatile growth hormone secretion is regulated.[25] The exact nature of this effect is dependent on the activating opioid compound.[26]
- Tolerance to morphine in part appears due to one of its metabolites, morphine-3-glucuronide, which has been shown to antagonise the ventilatory depressant and analgesic effects of both morphine and morphine-6-glucuronide. It is also believed that morphine-3-glucuronide is responsible for the hyperalgesia, allodynia, and myoclonus seen following high-dose morphine administration.[27]
- Morphine pharmacokinetics which are altered in the critically ill. A reduced volume of distribution for both morphine and lignocaine has been demonstrated. Lignocaine clearance was found to be normal in these patients, while morphine clearance was reduced, suggesting that alterations in hepatic blood flow were not responsible for the reduction in morphine clearance as had previously been believed.[28]

The examples given above are of predictable drug actions. But what of the unpredictable drug actions? These are actions that are unrelated to the known pharmacology of the drug, not related to drug tissue concentrations, and that carry a higher mortality risk than predictable reactions. Examples might include electrolyte and fluid balance abnormalities after carbamazepine therapy, pulmonary fibrosis secondary to practolol, aplastic anaemia with chlorpromazine treatment, and hepatitis induced by non-steroidal anti-inflammatory drugs.

Practicalities of patient care in the critically ill

Simple measures, such as the adequate labelling of intravenous infusion pumps, syringes, and lines, can reduce the risks of inadvertent errors of drug administration, particularly in emergency situations. Critically ill patients often have a multitude of infusion pumps and lines, and it is all too easy to adjust the rate of the wrong infusion pump, or mix incompatible infusions through the same line. Many units employ standard dilutions of drugs used frequently, including inotropes, which again reduces the risks of errors of drug calculation and dosage.

Most ICUs cover arterial lines with a labelled dressing, and use colour-coded pressure-transducing lines with a single, coloured, three-way tap for sampling, to reduce the risk of inadvertent intra-arterial injection of drugs. Inclusion of more than one three-way tap in an arterial circuit not only results in damping of the trace, but it also increases the risks of intra-arterial drug administration with all its attendant complications.

No matter how detailed the knowledge about drugs, unless doctors can communicate their intended prescription to colleagues clearly, drug errors will be made, and patients will suffer the consequences. The earliest recorded written prescription is contained in the Ebers Papyrus,[29] an Egyptian medical compendium dating back to about 1550 BC. Ever since then, prescribing has been fraught with many dangers and pitfalls. To reduce the risks of mistakes with drug administrations:

- Prescriptions should be written legibly, in block capital letters, using approved drug names.
- All prescriptions should include the date the treatment is prescribed.
- All prescriptions should be reviewed each day – patient circumstances change, and what were appropriate treatments and doses yesterday may be inappropriate today.
- Drug doses should be carefully considered for the circumstances of each individual patient.
- All treatment charts should include, in a prominent place, a statement of any known drug allergies to be completed and signed by the doctor initiating drug treatment. If there are no known drug allergies, this statement should be included and signed.
- For treatments of a specified duration, a stop date should always be entered in the drug chart. This is especially important for antibiotics, where the prescription should also include the indication for the antibiotic, for example, chest infection, urinary tract infection.
- Where intravenous drugs are to be administered as a bolus, they should be given through peripheral venous access, to minimise the potential risk of introducing infection via the central venous access by repeated connection and disconnection of syringes and infusion-giving sets.
- For all drug infusions, it must be confirmed that the drug and its intended carrier solution are compatible.
- All possible routes of drug administration should be considered. It is important to remember that gastrointestinal absorption in the critically ill can be very variable, and that subcutaneous and intramuscular routes have variable absorption in hypoperfusional states. The rectal route is often overlooked, but usually offers rapid and predictable absorption. Other routes of drug administration, including transdermal, transbuccal, inhalational, epidural, and spinal, should not be overlooked, particularly in the case of analgesic prescriptions.

- No prescription should be altered in any way. If changes need to be made, the original prescription should be crossed off, with a signature, and the new prescription written out again in full.
- Where available, information about possible drug interactions should be sought before initiating any new therapy. Sources could include a pharmacist, a computer programme, a National Formulary, or the Internet.
- Finally, if you are still in any doubt, don't prescribe without asking.

1 *British National Formulary Number 37.* London: British Medical Association, 1999. pp 1,244.
2 Paw HGW, Park GR. *Drug prescribing in anaesthesia and intensive care.* Oxford: Oxford University Press, 1996. pp 73,60–61.
3 Omoigui S. *The anaesthesia drugs handbook,* 2nd edn. St Louis: Mosby, 1995. pp 1–3, 354–7.
4 Hope RA, Longmore JM. *Oxford handbook of clinical medicine.* Oxford: Oxford Medical Publications, 1985. p 246.
5 Read AE, Barritt DW, Langton Hewer R. *Modern medicine,* 3rd edn. London: Pitman Publishing, 1984. p 315.
6 Aitkenhead AR, Smith G. *Textbook of anaesthesia,* 2nd edn. Edinburgh: Churchill Livingstone, 1990. pp 345, 438.
7 Association of the British Pharmaceutical Industry. *Compendium of patient information leaflets.* London: Datapharm Publications, 1994. p 67.
8 Stoelting RK. *Pharmacology and physiology in anesthetic practice,* 2nd edn. Philadelphia: JB Lippincott, 1991: 24.
9 Hill JB. Salicylate Intoxication. *N Engl J Med* 1973;**288**:1110–13.
10 Chernow B. *The pharmacologic approach to the critically ill patient,* 2nd edn. Baltimore: Williams & Wilkins, 1988.
11 Reidenberg MM, Affrime M. Influence of disease on binding of drugs to plasma proteins. *Ann N Y Acad Sci* 1973;**226**:115–26.
12 Bachmann K, Shapiro R, Mackiewicz J. Influence of renal dysfunction on warfarin plasma protein binding. *J Clin Pharmacol* 1976;**16**:468–72.
13 Brewster D, Muir NC. Valproate plasma protein binding in the uraemic condition. *Clin Pharmacol Ther* 1980;**27**:76–82.
14 Bevan JA, Thompson JH. *Essentials of pharmacology,* 3rd edn. Philadelphia: Harper and Row, 1983: 855.
15 Aronson JK. Clinical pharmacokinetics of digoxin. *Clin Pharmacokinet* 1980;**5**:137–49.
16 Murphy MR, Hugg CC, McClain DD. Dose-dependent pharmacokinetics of fentanyl. *Anesthesiology* 1983;**59**:537–40.
17 Don HF, Dieppa RD, Taylor P. Narcotic analgesics in anuric patients. *Anesthesiology* 1975;**42**:745–7.
18 Hoke JF, Shlugman D, Dershwitz M *et al.* Pharmacokinetics and pharmacodynamics of remifentanil in persons with renal failure compared with healthy volunteers. *Anesthesiology* 1997;**87**:533–41.
19 Webster NR. Opioids and the immune system. *Br J Anaesth* 1998;**81**:835–6.
20 Chang SL, Wu GD, Patel NA, Vidal EL, Fiala M. The effects of interaction between morphine and interleukin-1 on the immune response. *Adv Exp Med Biol* 1998;**437**:67–72.
21 Mellon RD, Bayer BM. Evidence for central opioid receptors in the immunomodulatory effects of morphine: review of potential mechanism(s) of action. *J Neuroimmunol* 1998;**83**:19–28.
22 Henrohn D, Le Greves P, Nyberg F. Morphine alters the level of growth hormone receptor mRNA and [125I] growth hormone binding in human IM-9 lymphoblasts via a naloxone-reversible mechanism. *Mol Cell Endocrinol* 1997;**135**:147–52.
23 Hashiguchi Y, Molina PE, Dorton S *et al.* Central opiate mu-receptor-mediated suppression of tissue protein synthesis. *Am J Physiol* 1997;**273**:R920–7.
24 Tomasi PA, Fanciulli G, Palermo M, Pala A, Demontis MA, Delitala G. Opioid-receptor blockade blunts growth hormone secretion induced by GH-releasing hormone in the human male. *Horm Metab Res* 1998;**30**:34–6.

25 Willoughby JO, Medvedev A. Opioid receptor activation resets the hypothalamic clock generating growth hormone secretory bursts in the rat. *J Endocrinol* 1996;**148**:149–55.
26 Hashiguchi Y, Molina PE, Fan J, Lang CH, Abumrad NN. Central opiate modulation of growth hormone and insulin-like growth factor-I. *Brain Res Bull* 1996;**40**:99–104.
27 Christrup LL. Morphine metabolites. *Acta Anaesthesiol Scand* 1997;**41**:116–22.
28 Berkenstadt H, Segal E, Mayan H *et al.* The pharmacokinetics of morphine and lidocaine in critically ill patients. *Intens Care Med* 1999;**25**:110–12.
29 Duin N, Sutcliffe J. *A history of medicine.* London: Readers Digest, 1992: 12.

Index

continuous enteral nutrition 120–1
Continus 171
contraceptive pill 174
contraindications 170–4
corticosteroids 80, 140–1
coumarin 46
covalent bonding 1–2
COX-1 37
COX-2 37
creatinine clearance 57, 74, 107
cyanide 80
cyclic 3, 5–adenosine monophosphate (cAMP) 44
cyclo-oxegenase 37
cyclosporin 12, 22, 31
cysteine 46
cystic fibrosis 147–8
cytochromes P450 21, 22, 24, 25, 26, 27, 28, 29, 51, 53, 92, 93, 94, 95, 108, 140, 152, 161, 162, 174
cytokines 24, 94, 117, 129

d-hyoscyamine 4
d-methyltubocurarine 64, 65
d-tubocurarine 3, 64, 65, 67
deaths, ICU patients 111
debrisoquine 29, 93
decarboxylase 6
dehydropeptidase-1 23, 31
depolarising neuromuscular relaxants 65
desacetyl metabolites 69
desmethyldiazepam 54
detection systems 12
dexamethasone 141
dextromethorphan O-demethylation 162
dextrorotatory enantiomer 2
dextrorphan 162
dextrose 127
diacylglycerol 44, 45
diafiltration 53
diazepam 5, 29, 50, 52, 54, 105, 133
diazoxide 38
didanosine 13
digitoxin 105
digoxin 12, 13, 78, 80, 104, 109, 111, 117, 148, 150, 151, 174
dihydrocodeine 59, 63, 64
dihydroketamine 52
diltiazem 80, 111
5–(1,3–dimethylbutyl)-5–ethyl barbituric acid 4
dipivaloyl 6
dipoles 2
direct enzyme-linked receptors 45
disopyramide 103

displacement, binding sites 18
diuretic theory 138
diuretics 37, 80, 81, 111, 141
dizocilpine 137
dobutamine 4, 26, 79–80, 111, 119
L-dopa (L-3,4–dihydroxyphenylalanine) 6
dopamine 79, 108, 119, 150
doperamine 119
dopexamine 80, 108, 119
dosage 177
doxacurium 64, 70
doxycycline 75
drug absorption 16–17
  age 158
  cardiac failure 103–4
  contraindications and side effects 171–2
  drug delivery 7
  from rectum 121
  gut failure 117
  hepatic failure 89–90
  respiratory failure 145–7, 150, 151
drug action 36–47
drug distribution 17–18
  age 158–60
  cardiac failure 104–5
  contraindications and side effects 172
  hepatic failure 90
  respiratory failure 147–8, 150, 151
drug elimination 20–8
  age 163
  contraindications and side effects 173–4
  hepatic 90–5, 107–9, 148
  renal 55–7, 105–7, 148
  respiratory failure 148–9, 150–1, 151–4
drug interactions 30–1
  absorption 171
  information on 178
  liver disease 95–6
drugs
  administration 177–8
  brain failure 125–42
  cardiac failure 102–11
  children 158–64
  contraindications 170–4
  defined 1–6
  formulations 6–10
  guidelines and protocols 170
  gut failure 114–22
  hepatic failure 28, 89–99
  indications 167–70

186

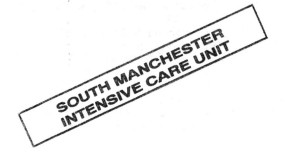

SOUTH MANCHESTER
INTENSIVE CARE UNIT